PRAYA

Cracking Homeopathic Codes
in
Breast Cancer

Dr Sunirmal Sarkar
Dr Shruti Shah

B. JAIN PUBLISHERS (P) LTD.
USA—Europe—India

Cracking Homeopathic Codes in Breast Cancer
First Edition: 2020
1st Impression: 2020

Published by Kuldeep Jain for
B. JAIN PUBLISHERS (P) LTD.
D-157, Sector-63, NOIDA-201307, U.P. (INDIA)
Tel.: +91-120-4933333 • *Email:* info@bjain.com
Website: **www.bjainbooks.com**
Registered office: 1921/10, Chuna Mandi, Paharganj,
New Delhi-110 055 (India)

Printed in India

ISBN: 978-81-319-1382-6

Inspiration And Blessings From
Shri Mahavatar Babaji

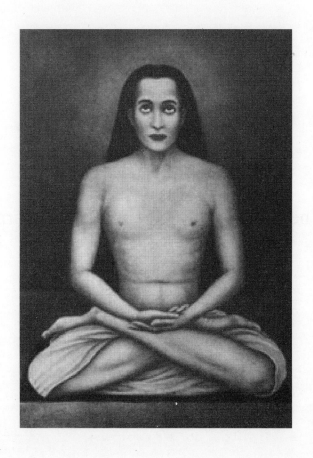

Dedicated To,
The One Who Really Wants To Learn.

Acknowledgement

First of all, I would like to thank the Almighty and my beloved Guru Shri Paramhansa Yoganandji for their eternal grace which is the driving force for me.

My father Dr Pravin Shah, Ph.D. has always remained such a powerful presence in my life. He taught me to learn, dream and believe in dreams. He himself is a scientist and has been my source of inspiration since childhood till today in all my endeavors. I am so much fortunate to have him as my father. My mother, Mrs. Pushpa Shah, is the physical form of grace I just mentioned about and this book would not have been finished without her support. She took care of home, kids when her crazy daughter was busy cracking some abstract codes.

My life partner, Dr Ritesh Jani, has thoroughly cooperated with me during writing breaks and has taken care of me always. I am lucky to have him with me as a companion.

My kids, Keya and Kishlay, who are running in their 16th year, are extremely exceptional they have sacrificed a lot for this book. This book from Mom has stolen share of their time and they have always understood and cooperated with a sweet complaint that this book has given lot of pain to us.

I got another parents duo after marriage, my in-laws, Mr. Narendra Jani and Mrs. Pushpa Jani, and I full-heartedly convey my thanks to them for their blessings and support. I am blessed to have a large family and I would like to thank each and every member for their love and support, especially Dr Tushar- Dr Niti Shah, Dr Manish-Dr Kshama Shah, Dr Akshay Jani, Dr Kalrav Joshi; Mr. Mahendra Shah, who is my uncle and manages my pharmacy, and Ms. Jaya Manwani, who has taken care of my family since years.

Dr Sunirmal Sarkar Sir has always taught me with so much love, and it is my immense pleasure to become a co-author of this book alongwith him.

I also want to convey my gratitude to Mr. Yunus Lakadia from Bhavnagar. He is not a doctor but an ardent learner of Homeopathy. He was my first teacher and a lifetime strong supporter.

Dr Kenali Kankotiya and Dr Shreya Sachapara, my students, have just finished their internship. I am really grateful to both of them for their immense support and hard work in this book. They are actually God sent angels who helped me to complete this book on time. My sister and colleague, Dr Hiral Shah, has also been instrumental, her laughter and wit have been of great service.

My dearest friends, Dr Hardik Khamar, Dr Vismay Thaker from Ahmedabad; Dr Shizuko Nagasawa of Japan; Dr Zahid Shah from Bhiwandi; Fons Vanderleyden from Belgium; Theresa Shriecke from Vienna; Hiral-Niraj Meghani, Chintan Vyas and Umesh-Dipti Shah from Bhavnagar, deserve a special thanks from the bottom of my heart. Hardik and Vismay have been partners in crime since the beginning of college days and thankfully they are still my partners throughout, since the conception of 'Prayas' till today. Umeshbhai has always been an enthusiastic supporter of all my wise and mad deeds and I convey my gratitude to him.

My housemaid and part of our family since last 11 years, Mrs. Jiluben, cannot be forgotten for her selfless love and care.

I am also thankful to Dr Srinivasulu Gadugu from Hyderabad for writing the foreword of this book and for his help in building me from a senior homoeopath to a novice researcher when I just started my research career.

I am immensely thankful to my school, Shri Daxinamoorti Vidyamandir, where I have spent the best years of my life, my teachers, schoolmates; my colleges, Ahmedabad Homoeopathic Medical College where I completed my BHMS and MD and Swami Vivekanand Homeopathic Medical College, where I completed my PhD and also work as a Lecturer; all the students and faculties who helped me to learn this wonderful art of Medicine; cannot forget to mention are Dr Jayesh Patel, Dr Ahalparasir, Dr Heena Rawal, Dr Vandana Shah, Dr Gayatri Anjariya, Dr Falguni Thakkar, Mrs. Shilpa Doshi (our librarian), Dr Ashish Mehta, Dr Apurva Patel and Dr Girish Patel.

I also want to thank all the homeopaths, doctors, scientists, researchers who have been working day and night to serve mankind and whose work has been the foundation of this book, author of all the books/research papers I have referred to as it is not been possible to mention all the names. Also, a big thanks to the makers of Mac Repertory, it has been such a useful tool. Special names I take with reverence from this community of learned men are Dr Samuel Hahnemann, Dr Arthur Hill Grimmer and Dr David Little, whose contribution to medical science/cancer therapy is incredible but has not been acknowledged enough. I would like to thank Dr Rajan Sankaran for his innovative teachings.

Dr Kenali, Dr Shreya, Dr Meera and Mr. Bhavyesh Acharya have worked together for the graphics and designing. Glossary given after the book has been prepared by Dr Shreya.

Dr Jinali Samani from Bhavnagar has enriched this book with her valuable suggestions.

Last but not least, my sincere thanks to all the Cancer patients who have come to me for treatment, they have been my best teachers and their spirit to fight till the last breath have taught me a lot.

Their faith in me and indomitable wish to live have inspired me to perfect my learning in Cancer therapy, and one of the results is this book.

I cannot forget to mention Mr. Manish Jain of B. Jain Publishers who actually gave me an idea to pen down my research work in the form of a book. I am grateful to him as well as the team of B. Jain Publishers.

Dr Shruti Shah,
Bhavnagar.

Why This Book?

Few years ago, a personal tragedy made me realizes that there is a very limited scope for cancer patients in the modern medicine. There are few treatment options which are full of side effects and after going through these side effects, most of the precious lives are lost.

My experience of treating few Cancer patients with Homeopathy made me fully convinced that there is tremendous potential for cancer treatment in Homeopathy. It made me study the application of Homeopathy for Cancer in detail. During my practice, I have studied almost all the literature available for Homeopathy and management of Cancer .

I discovered a Gold Mine for Cancer treatment in Homeopathic Science. I began with a small charitable clinic offering Homeopathic treatment to Cancer patients, exactly 5 years ago. As the work grew, I happened to meet and learn from Respected Dr Sarkar which resulted in the foundation of "Prayas Homeopathy and Cancer Research Foundation" along with my colleagues Dr Hardik Khamar, Dr Ritesh Jani, Dr Shizuko Nagasawa, Dr Vismay Thaker, and Dr Kausha Khamar. 'Prayas' has always aimed to offer standardized Homeopathic treatment to Cancer patients and promote research activities in the same field. Till now, Prayas holds four Cancer OPD's affiliated with it in India.

Setting up was an easy task but treating patients with grave pathologies came out to be most difficult. I am really fortunate to have Dr Sarkar as my mentor and getting an opportunity to learn from him in his own OPD where he sees thousands of Cancer patients.

Again, results do mesmerise, and gaining knowledge was easy but to reproduce the same standard of results in my own OPD was the bigger task. I have often envied Dr Sarkar's Grey Matter, Neurons, their Inner Connections silently, and sometimes even publicly.

I studied Cancer Specific Remedies mentioned by Dr Grimmer after seeing Dr Sarkar applying them very successfully in his clinic. But it is challenging to differentiate between lesser known Cancer Remedies when a virgin cancer case approaches to a Homeopath opting for Homeopathy as a sole treatment option or a patient with secondary cancer already spread in the body's entire system with no other option left for him.

Gold Mine of Cancer Remedies lies in very crude form, still left to be dig and got polished. It's all scattered in various source books, clinical Materia Medica, documented clinical experiences and cases, repertories, but was not updated and integrated with the modern science which made its application much challenging.

When I look for the current research of our well-known cancer remedies, I discovered that almost every medicine was proven for its efficacy for cancer in the form of alcoholic or crude extract by various scientists of varied fields. There is plethora of information about their clinical indications, phytochemistry, molecular biology, pathways they affect and detailed pathology produced or cured by them. But these latest findings are not integrated with our Materia Medica which makes application of these remedies limited and also making it difficult for the modern doctors to relate to our Pharmacology.

Hence, I took up studying the current findings of our Cancer Remedies and integrated them with our Materia Medica to make our remedies more applicable. I had to study 200 to 500, sometimes around 1000 research papers, and various source books to conclude the molecular or biochemical actions of each Cancer Remedy relevant to a Homeopath.

It was still a theoretical aspect when I started studying Homeopathic Literature under the guidance of Dr Sarkar, a man who knows how to practically apply the information available in clinic with success. According to his guidance and experience, from various Homeopathic textbooks, I extracted the most required symptoms to prescribe.

The Homeopathic Masters referred to pick up noteworthy symptoms of Materia Medica includes Dr Grimmer, Dr T.F. Allen, Dr Bernoville, Dr Boericke, Dr Clarke, Dr Knerr, Dr Samuel Lilienthal and Dr Pulford.

51 remedies are listed under Breast Cancer in Kent's Repertory and more than 200 in Complete Repertory, out of which I selected the most important and lesser known ones.

Thus, this Materia Medica of Breast Cancer (Oncology Materia Medica) is prepared including more than 80 Breast Cancer Remedies. It includes olden golden experience of our Homeopathic Masters and is integrated with the latest findings.

The book aims to make prescribing for breast cancer easy by bringing all the scattered information at one place in order to make the task easier for our fellow physicians .

The anther motive is to bring more awareness about Homeopathy and its potential role in the management of Cancer.

This book can also be used as a guide or map while treating Breast Cancer.

I have also included a brief description about the Clinical Approach to be followed while dealing with Cancer Patients.

I am glad to present this work to the whole medical fraternity. I pray to *the Almighty* that it may serve as a useful tool for our medical colleagues, and helps to enhance the research work and reduce the sufferings due to "Deadly Cancer - The Emperor Of All Maladies".

This Book is a humble "EFFORT" to combine contemporary medicine and classical homoeopathic medicine for the goodness of mankind.

Dr Shruti Shah

Publisher's Note

This book, "Cracking The Homeopathic Codes In Breast Cancer" by Dr Sunirmal Sarkar and Dr Shruti Shah, covers everything one needs to know to empower while dealing with cases of Breast Cancer, and is packed full of remedies that prove to be useful in such cases.

The book is based on the authentic literature as well as the clinical experience of Dr Sunirmal Sarkar, one of the Homeopathic Experts, and will help the readers to gain an understanding about the indications of various medicines that can be employed in different cases of Breast Cancer. Each remedy is segregated according to its kingdom and the accurate symptoms are described aptly under the medicine. The authors have tried their level best to cover the remedies from all kingdoms such as plant, animal and mineral, as well as from nosodes, sarcodes, radioactive substances, synthetic sources, and few of the new plant remedies. We are thankful to the Editor, Dr Yashika Arora, for her tireless and speedy efforts to bring out the book in its best form.

It is a valuable read for Homeopaths involved in the care of patients suffering from Breast Cancer, the most common form of cancer in women, and is completely dispassionate to age, race, and ethnicity. We hope that this work, providing an insight to

Materia Medica, proves to be a great resource for the homeopathic physicians while treating the patients of Breast Cancer.

Kuldeep Jain
CEO, B. Jain Publishers (P) Ltd.

Contents

Acknowledgement .... *v*

Why This Book? .... *ix*

Publisher's Note .... *xiii*

1. Breast Cancer: Its Clinical Aspects 1

2. Clinical Approach in Breast Cancer 11

3. Homeopathic Remedies for Breast Cancer 19

4. Plant Remedies 25

5. Animal Remedies 83

6. Mineral Remedies... 113

7. Nosodes 135

8. Sarcodes... 139

9. Radioactive Substances 155

10. Synthetic Remedies 161

11. New Plant Remedies For Cancer............................ 169

Glossary *185*

Bibliography *195*

Chapter 1

Breast Cancer: Its Clinical Aspects

Introduction

Cancer is defined as a group of diseases which involves abnormal cell growth with the potential to invade or spread to other parts of the body.

In 2015, about 90.5 million people suffered from Cancer, about 14.1 million new cases resulted in that year which caused around 8.8 million deaths (15.7% of deaths).

As per 2010 census, the financial costs of Cancer were estimated at $1.16 trillion USD per year.

It is one of the most challenging and dreadful diseases causing extreme human sufferings, morbidity and financial loss.

Causes of Cancer

Cancer has a multifactorial pathology and it requires a number of years along with a series of accidents/events for a cancer cell to develop and turn into a malignant growth. Though no definite cause for cancer is known yet, but there are certainly few factors which are found to be associated with it as follows:

1. Heredity-DNA: Cancer can be a genetic disorder arising out of Abnormal Mutations in the Healthy Genome, which passes from generation to generation.

There are few types of Cancers which are strongly associated with the Family History.

2. Exposure to Carcinogens: Malignancy can also be associated with exposure to Carcinogens like Tobacco, Radioactive Emissions, and certain Chemicals, etc. These substances mutate or promote the abnormally mutated genes to multiply and thus initiating or hastening the process of Carcinogenesis.

3. Microbes: Certain Retroviruses, Bacteria and Fungi are also known to produce chronic inflammatory conditions which later on may turn into Cancer. For example, HPV causing Cervical and Oral Cancer, Helicobacterium Pylori leading to Stomach Cancer.

4. Psychological Factors: Psychological Factors like Emotional Trauma, Prolonged Grief, Stress, Disturbed Mental Environment for long, etc. may also lead to development of deeper pathologies like Cancer.

Breast Cancer

Breast cancer is defined as malignant proliferation of epithelial cells lining the ducts or lobules of the breast.

Causes: Epithelial malignancies of the breast are the most common causes of cancer in women.

Lifetime risk: 12.28%; 1 in 8 women.

Risk factors

1. Aging
2. Inability to bear a Child (Infertility) or Breastfeed
3. Increase in level of certain Hormones
4. Dietary patter
5. Obesity
6. Alcohol intake
7. Use of Hormonal Birth Control Pills

8. Disruption of Biological Rhythm and Shift work
9. Exposure to Carcinogenic Substances
10. Exposure to Radiation
11. Certain Medical Conditions such as Fibrocystic Breast Disease and Lupus Erythematosus

Genetic consideration of Breast Cancer

To some extent, Breast Cancer can be hereditary in nature. The BRCA genes are the tumor suppressor genes which prevent uncontrolled cell growth and abnormal cells turning into cancerous. The harmful mutations in these BRCA 1 and BRCA 2 genes may produce a "Heredity Ovarian Breast Cancer Syndrome" in the affected individuals. Such women may have five times higher risk of Breast Cancer, and about ten to thirty times higher risk of ovarian cancer than normal women. Mutations can be inherited from either parent and may pass on to son or daughter both. BRCA-related breast cancer appears at an earlier age than sporadic breast cancer. It has been asserted that BRCA-related Breast Cancer is more aggressive than normal Breast Cancer. These mutated genes are also associated with triple-negative Breast Cancer, which does not respond to hormonal treatment or any other drug.

Classification of Breast Cancer

1. Histopathological classification

1. DUCTAL CARCINOMA IN-SITU: Its a non-invasive Breast Cancer in which abnormal cells are present in the lining of breast milk duct.
2. INVASIVE DUCTAL CARCINOMA (IDC): In IDC, abnormal cells originating in the lining of breast milk duct invades the surrounding tissues.

3. TRIPLE NEGATIVE BREAST CANCER: Triple negative breast cancer (TNBC) is clinically characterized by lack of expression of Estrogen, Progesterone and HER2 hormone receptors. It does not respond to the hormonal therapy (such as tamoxifen or aromatase inhibitors) or therapies that target HER2 receptors, such as Herceptin due to which women diagnosed with TNBC generally face a poorer prognosis.

4. INFLAMMATORY BREAST CANCER: This is a less common form where tumor develop over the skin. In inflammatory Breast Cancer, the cancer cells invade local lymphatic ducts, thus impairing drainage and causing edematous swelling of the breast.

5. PEAU D'ORANGE: In this, the skin of the breast is tethered by the suspensory ligament of Cooper, with the accumulation of fluid, which causes the breast to take a dimpled appearance similar to an orange.

6. METASTATIC BREAST CANCER: When the Cancer spreads beyond the breast, into lungs, bones or brain, it is termed as Metastatic Breast Cancer.

7. MEDULLARY CARCINOMA: It is a rare subtype of IDC that begins in the milk duct and spreads beyond it.

8. TUBULAR CARCINOMA: It is a sub-type of IDC with a low incidence of lymph node involvement and a high survival rate.

9. MUCINOUS CARCINOMA: It is also called colloid carcinoma, a rare form of IDC in which the cancerous cells produce mucus.

10. PAGET'S DISEASE OF BREAST OR NIPPLE: It is a cancer with an outward appearance of eczema along with skin changes involving the nipple of the breast. It is a chronic, eczematous eruption of nipple or breast which may progress to an ulcerated, weeping lesion.

2. Gradation as per Pathology

1. Well differentiated (low-grade) malignant cells
2. Moderately differentiated (intermediate grade) malignant cells
3. Poorly differentiated (high-grade) malignant cells
   The poorly differentiated cancerous cells have the worst prognosis.

3. Staging

The TNM classification for staging Breast Cancer is based on the size of Cancer, its origin in the body and sites involved.

The characteristics described include the size of the tumor (T), whether the tumor has spread to the lymph nodes (N) in the armpits, neck, and inside the chest, and whether the tumor has metastasized (M) (i.e. spread to a more distant part of the body).

The main stages include:

1. Stage 0: In-situ disease or Paget's disease of the nipple. It is a pre-cancerous or marker condition. For example: Ductal Carcinoma in Situ (DCIS) or Lobular Carcinoma in Situ (LCIS).
2. Stage 1 to Stage 3 are located within the breast or involve regional lymph nodes.
3. Stage 4 is the metastatic cancer having a less favorable prognosis.

Larger size, more nodal spread, and more number of sites metastasized possess the worst prognosis.

4. Classification based on the Receptor Status

Chemical messengers such as hormones bind to receptors present on the surface of cells, or inside the cytoplasm and nucleus, which causes changes in the cell. The three most important receptors include:

1. Estrogen Receptor (ER).
2. Progesterone Receptor (PR).
3. Herceptin Receptor (Her2/Neu) [Human Epidermal Growth Factor Receptor 2 is a cell membrane surface bound receptor normally involved in signal transduction pathways, cell growth and differentiation. 30% of breast cancers occur due to overexpression of its protein product].

The cancer cells may be classified as:

1. Cells with or without Estrogen receptor are called ER positive (ER+), ER negative (ER-).
2. Cells with or without Progesterone receptor are known as PR positive (PR+), PR negative (PR-).
3. Cells with or without Herceptin receptor are termed as HER2 positive (HER2+), and HER2 negative (HER2-).
4. Cells with none of these receptors are called Basal-like or Triple Negative cells.

5. DNA-based classification

In a cancerous cell, DNA or RNA testing is done by employing several different laboratory approaches. Identification of specific DNA mutations or gene expression profiles in the cancerous cells guides to the selection of treatment.

Signs and Symptoms of Breast Cancer

Symptoms of Breast Tumor vary from person to person and include:

1. Skin changes such as swelling, redness, or other visible differences in one or both breasts.
2. Increase in size or change in shape of the breast(s).

3. Change in the appearance of one or both nipples.
4. Nipple discharge other than breast milk.
5. General pain in/on any part of the breast.
6. Lump formation or nodes felt on or inside of the breast.

Symptoms more specific to invasive breast cancer are as follows:

1. Irritated or itchy breasts.
2. Change in breast color.
3. Increase in breast size or shape (over a short period of time).
4. Hard, tender or warm to touch.)
5. Peeling or flaking of the nipple's skin.
6. A lump or thickening in breast.
7. Redness or pitting of the breast skin (like the skin of an orange).

Diagnosis

Clinical	1. Age and risk factors 2. Examination: CBE(Clinical breast examination) and SBE(Self breast examination)
Imaging	1. Ultrasonography scan (USG) 2. Magnetic resonance imaging (MRI) 3. Mammography 4. Positron emission tomography scan (PET) 5. Scintimammography 6. Doppler flow studies 7. Thermography
Pathological	1. Fine needle aspiration cytology (FNAC) 2. Core cut needle biopsy

Management

Conventional treatment include

1. Surgery
2. Chemotherapy
3. Hormonal therapy
4. Radiation therapy
5. Cancer Vaccines (which are over the horizon)

Surgery

1. Breast-conserving surgery (BSC), also known as lumpectomy or wide local excision, involves resection of the tumor along with a margin of tissue while conserving the cosmetic appearance of the breast. Most breast surgeries are breast-conserving because most of the tumors are locally invasive, and also the large primary tumors can be reduced in size by neoadjuvant chemotherapy prior to conservative surgery.

2. Mastectomy is defined as surgical removal of entire breast including the fascia over the pectoralis muscles. Surgeons may preserve some skin and the nipple/areola for reconstruction. The indication for mastectomy is multicentric invasive carcinoma, inflammatory carcinoma, or extensive intraductal carcinoma.

3. Axillary lymph node dissection involves removal of the lymph nodes draining the breast tissue for lymph node micro metastasis, similar to BSC or mastectomy. However, recent evidences suggest that axillary lymph node biopsy is unnecessary regardless of whether the sentinel lymph node biopsy is negative or positive as there is no mortality benefit.

4. Adjuvant therapy like cytotoxic chemotherapy, endocrine therapy, or radiation therapy may be used post-surgery to prevent relapse.

Radiation Therapy

Breast irradiation, either whole or partial breast irradiation is applied. Adjuvant radiation therapy is applied post-BCS or post-mastectomy to prevent recurrence.

Conventionally, Radiotherapy is done after surgery to the region of the tumor bed and regional lymph nodes, in order to destroy microscopic tumor cells that may have escaped surgery. It can be delivered as external beam radiotherapy or as brachytherapy (internal radiotherapy). Radiation can also be given at the time of operating the Breast Cancer which may reduce the risk of recurrence by 50–66% (1/2 to 2/3 reduction of risk) when delivered in the correct dose.

Hormonal Therapy

Breast cancer is a hormone-sensitive cancer and some of the Breast Cancers require Estrogen to continue their growth. These ER+ cancers can be treated with drugs that may either block the receptors, e.g. tamoxifen; or alternatively block the production of Estrogen with an aromatase inhibitor, e.g. anastrozole or letrozole. The therapies include Ovarian ablation, Adrenalectomy, or Ovarian suppression (LHRH (GnRH) agonist (e.g. Goserelin and Leuprorelin) may be used to reversibly suppress LH/FSH release, thus estrogen release as well).

Chemotherapy

Chemotherapy is predominantly useful in Stage 2 to Stage 4 of breast cancer, and particularly beneficial in Estrogen receptor-negative (ER-) disease.

Medications in chemotherapy are administered in combinations, usually for a period of 3 to6 months. One of the most common regimens known as "AC" combines cyclophosphamide with doxorubicin.

Sometimes, a Taxene drug such as docetaxel may be added, and the regime is then known as "CAT".

Another common treatment used include cyclophosphamide, methotrexate, and fluorouracil (or "CMF").

Most of the medications given in chemotherapy work by destroying fast-growing and/or fast-replicating cancer cells, either by causing DNA damage or by other mechanisms. However, the medications also damage fast-growing normal cells leading to more serious side effects. Damage to the heart muscle is the most dangerous complication of doxorubicin.

Prevention

Women with breast cancer have 0.5% per year risk of developing a second breast cancer. But women at increased risk of breast cancer, can reduce their risk by 49% by consuming tamoxifen or an aromatase inhibitor for 5 years. Women with BRCA-1 mutations can also reduce the risk by 90% with simple mastectomy.

Chapter 2

Clinical Approach in Breast Cancer

Generally, no panacea or single remedy can cure a complex pathology like Breast Cancer.

Treating Breast Cancer with Homeopathy is seriously a challenging task requiring extreme carefulness, agility, clinical skills, and a series of remedies according to the patients' stage and presenting symptoms.

When a Cancer patient comes to a Homeopath's office, it can be in any stage with varied clinical presentations. A general outline of various clinical approaches to be opted while dealing with a Cancer case is discussed below. These are based on principles of Homeopathy and authors' own clinical experience.

Precancerous Breast Lesions

In Precancerous Breast Lesions, homoeopathic remedies prove to be very effective.

As a Homeopath, one needs to perform a detailed case taking first including patient's physical make-up, mental traits as well general likings related to food, atmosphere and peculiarities of physiological and psychological functions, which helps to determine the Constitutional Remedy.

Mostly, a well-selected Constitutional Remedy with a judicious use of respective Nosode helps to clear the lesion, thus preventing it from becoming cancerous further.

Primary Cancer

Cases with Primary Cancer are the most challenging and the most fruitful ones for a Homeopath.

Mostly, the patients go for surgery, chemotherapy and radiation, and then prefer Homeopathy along with or afterwards.

In each case, the following parameters need to be investigated:

1. Any emotional grief, mental trauma prior to development of cancer
2. History of Injury to breast
3. History of Lactation
4. History of taking Hormonal pills
5. History of Menstruation, Pregnancy and Abortion, if any
6. Addictions, if any
7. Exposure to Carcinogens
8. Past History
9. Family Medical History and medical history of Spouse as well
10. Detailed Case-Taking

One must remember the following words before beginning with the case:

" NOTHING HAPPENS, IF NOTHING HAPPENS."

Unresolved mental trauma, emotional conflicts, prolonged stress may pave way to Carcinogenesis in a fertile soil, infected with miasmatic pollutants. One must understand the cause and treat with a suitable homeopathic remedy to complete the Cure.

Guidelines to be followed:

A Cancer Case rarely yields a single indicated remedy. Generally, a series of well-chosen remedies are required to accomplish the cure along with the strategies mentioned below:

1. Firstly, the issue need to be addressed on the surface, and then layer by layer up to the core. Thus, managing the cancer case with a series of indicated homeopathic remedies, one after another, has been found to be the most successful strategy during clinical practice.

2. The factors which precipitated malignancy need to be antidoted along with Constitutional Remedy (CR), Nosode as well as a remedy according to local pathology to drain the toxins as per requirement of the case.

3. The general rule is to provide CR and Nosode in high potency, pathological remedy in low potency and drainage remedy in Q. Using dilution methods of LM potency/ ascending potency/plussing potency are found to shorten the duration required for cure, limiting the risk of giving a dry dose in higher potency.

4. If patient is taking Chemotherapy or Radiation, suitable remedies, at times, are needed to nullify the side effects.

5. Advice avoidance of factors contributing to the Malignancy along with balanced diet, counselling and lifestyle changes.

6. Many a times, there can be a paucity of symptoms and only local pathology may be prominent. To prescribe in such a case, the below mentioned factors can be considered:

   a. Sensation

   b. Modalities

   c. Concomitant symptoms/pathologies

   d. Type of Carcinoma (anatomical/histopathological)

   e. System and organ to which metastasis has taken place

Secondary Cancer with Metastasis

Secondary Cancer cases with Metastasis are comparatively difficult to treat due to poor vitality, paucity of symptoms and severe side effects of conventional cancer therapies.

In such patients, the primary prescription is based on pathology, good drainage and nullification of side effects.

Also, to improve patients' vitality, advice special nutrition, detoxification and counselling.

Later on, a good constitutional remedy or a nosode preferably in LM potency may be prescribed which gives a hard battle to the termed "INCURABLES".

Homeopathic Prevention

The Patient with no past history of Cancer but with a strong family history of Cancer.

For example, the famous Hollywood actress, Angelina Jolly, underwent Total Mastectomy for preventing the recurrence.

But such cases are many a times, positive for BRCA gene mutation.

In this scenario, a suitable Nosode with Constitutional Remedy prove to be of great help.

Note: In cases with past history of Cancer but presenting with no symptoms, Nosode and CR play an utmost role along with regular follow up, keen observation, regular assessment for biomarkers. These are mandatory as such patients can go into relapse anytime.

A detailed study with good statistics is required to prove the efficacy of Homeopathic therapy as it is frequently observed that Homeopathy proves to be very successful in preventing the relapse or giving a longer progression free survival time to the patients with past history of cancer.

Role of Homeopathy in management of the side effects of conventional therapy

Homeopathy also proves to be useful in combating the adverse reactions caused due to aggressive cancer therapies the patient undergo.

These include:

1. Hairfall
2. Cachexia
3. Leukopenia, Anemia, Thrombocytopenia
4. Hypoproteinemia
5. Gastrointestinal disturbances
6. Radiation Burns
7. Non-healing Ulcers and Wounds
8. Post-surgical complications
9. Psychosis, Mental Trauma, Anxiety and Fear
10. Depression, Suicidal tendencies, etc.
11. Secondary Cancer

There are numerous remedies in Materia Medica to treat the side effects of Chemotherapy, Radiation and Surgical complications effectively.

Homeopathic Palliation

Sometimes, as in incurable or fairly advanced cancer cases, merely passing the remaining days of life with minimum pain and maximum ease is the only option available. The agony in such cases is sometimes terrible as it is the terminal stage. These cases are generally seen during the initial phase of practice and require dedication and knowledge to relieve the agony.

Homeopathic remedies are effective to sooth the last days and can be used frequently.

Severe Malnutrition and Cachexia

Most of the Cancer patients suffer with malnutrition as the malignant cells keep on growing at the cost of healthy cells. Many a times, conventional therapies also contribute by depleting the healthy cells and fluids while killing the malignant cells aggressively.

Cancer cases do require nutritional diet, detoxification as well addition of anti-cancer food.

The indicated homeopathic remedy covering the symptoms of Cachexia can also be administered along, if the symptoms are severe.

Conclusion

Thus, there shall be no rigidity or fixity in clinical approach.

One must remember, "To prescribe ably on what patient demands by the most intense presenting symptoms is the key to success. For example, if local symptoms are characteristically stronger, pathology should be the base of prescription. If there is mental trauma or symptomatology overshadowing, a remedy covering the same needs to be given. When there is strong heredity or the constitutional symptoms are loud, the prescription should be based accordingly. If a patient chooses to go into his innermost sensation spontaneously, that approach should be taken up. So, it may be likewise according to the presenting situation. A patient is the one who decides what shall be the clinical approach and the physician learns the art to flow with the naturally presented stream of totality."

A Short Sample of Case Taking of Cancer patients

Name:

Age:

Sex:

Profession:

Marital Status:

Address:

Phone Number:

Diagnosis:

Chief Complaints:

- Location, Sensation, Modalities, Concomitants:
- Origin, Duration and Progress of Disease:

Past Medical History:

Family Medical History:

Personal History:

- Appetite
- Craving
- Aversion
- Thirst
- Habit or Addiction
- Bowel Habits
- Urinary System
- Perspiration
- Thermals
- Reaction to Hunger

- Reaction to Motion
- Reaction to Closed Room
- Reaction to Tight clothing
- Sleep; patient's position or abnormal behaviors/patterns during sleep
- Dreams
- Fear and Phobia
- Strong Mental/Emotional/Will symptoms; as narrated by patient, relatives as well as observed by physician
- Menstrual and Gynecological/Obstetric History
- Sexual Life

Note:

A Physician must record the whole case according to his clinical findings and observations.

Chapter 3

Homeopathic Remedies for Breast Cancer

There are 51 remedies listed under Breast Cancer in *Kent's Repertory* while more than 200 remedies mentioned in *Complete Repertory*.

Few of these remedies, especially the known constitutional ones, helps to strengthen the system for Precancerous or Post-cancerous stage of Cancer. Cancer specific remedies described later in this chapter are based on the pathology itself and can be prescribed during the active stage of disease as per the indications. But one must prescribe following the Law of Similia in each case to result in cure of the sick.

The well-known constitutional homeopathic remedies for Breast Cancer include:

1. Aconitum napellus
2. Alumina
3. Apis mellifica
4. Arnica montana
5. Argentum nitricum
6. Arsenicums'
7. Aurum metallicum
8. Baptisia tinctoria
9. Barytas'

10. Belladonna

11. Bromides'

12. Bryonia alba

13. Calcareas'

14. Carbons'

15. Chamomilla

16. Cicuta virosa

17. Colocynthis

18. Corydalis formosa

19. Cuprum metallicum

20. Eucalyptus

21. Ferrum metallicum

22. Ferrum iodatum

23. Fluorides'

24. Formicum acidum

25. Formalin

26. Bacillus Gartner

27. Hepar sulphuricum

28. Hippuric acidum

29. Hippozaenium

30. Ignatia amara

31. Iodides'

32. Kali salts

33. Lachesis mutus

34. Lapis album

35. Lycopodium clavatum

36. Magnesium carbonicum

37. Medorrhinum

38. Mercurius
39. Natrum carbonicum
40. Nitricum acidum
41. Pulsatilla nigricans
42. Oxalicum acidum
43. Phosphoricum acidum
44. Phosphorus
45. Platina
46. Psorinum
47. Rhus toxicodendron
48. Ruta graveolens
49. Sepia officinalis
50. Silicea/Silicates'
51. Sulphur
52. Staphysagria
53. Tarentula hispanica
54. Tuberculinum
55. Thuja occidentalis
56. Zincum metallicum

Some of these homeopathic remedies are explained in the further chapters. Some of them are omitted as they are found to be more indicated for intermittent stage of Cancer than Malignancy itself, they are very well-known or not strongly indicated.

The same goes for other medicines as well which are not mentioned in this book but can be the indicated at any given moment, if the symptoms call for.

Since there cannot be any rigid or fixed protocol, a flexibility in practice with open mindedness to prescribe as per the need of the moment, is the key for successful prescription.

Breast Cancer Specific Remedies

In the coming chapters, the main Breast Cancer Specific Remedies, grouped as per their source of origin, are described with their sphere of action and main indications.

All these remedies are recognized and proven for their anti-cancer properties by Homeopathic stalwarts. In fact, the modern cancer scientists and researchers too have recognized the definite anti-cancer role of these drugs in their separate experiments, due to which an in-depth research has also been carried out for most of them.

In spite of their proven efficacy, these medicines are not used extensively due to the following reasons:

1. Many Homeopathic doctors have done a significantly incredible work in Cancer treatment from Dr Ely G. Jones, Dr Burnett, Dr John Henry Clarke, Dr William Cooper, Dr Arthur Hill Grimmer to the current physicians like Dr P. Banerjee, Dr Ramakrishnan, Dr Alok Pareek, Dr Farokh Master, Dr Sunirmal Sarkar and many more.

2. This was being carried out on individual scale, but no strong system has been erected to carry it forward on the larger scale till now.

3. Due to lack of a standardized protocol for Homeopathic Treatment of Cancer and paucity of relevant textbooks related to particular pathology or disease, it requires superhuman caliber to master the art of homeopathic prescription in complex pathologies .

4. The remedies described are still in the language of old school, and not integrated with the current findings or expressed in new terminologies which makes it difficult for the non-homeopaths and scientists to correlate.

5. Homeopathic medicines have insufficient evidences in cancer management for its efficacy to be accepted as the reliable

method of treatment, according to the need of the modern standards and parameters.

6. There is no bridge which connects the gap between the Modern Medicine and the Homeopathy.

7. There are so many evidences of the natural plant and animal remedies for their anti-cancer roles. To prescribe them in harmless but effective doses and their availability poses a big challenge. Modern scientists are unaware of the revolutionary methods of drug dilution and potentization which helps to make a drug more potent harnessing side effects of its crude form . For example, anti-cancer potential of Cobra venom is established in modern medicine, but they are still unaware of how to give it without side effects, how to prevent it from getting digested by gastric juices and also how to meet the needs of the market without harming the natural resources. Homeopathic Science is a solution to it, but the world is not fully aware of it yet.

8. The modern medicine is still struggling to develop real cure, which is only possible using a Genetic Remedy. While Dr Hahnemann has already done it years ago by giving the most powerful tools of Individualized Constitutional Remedy and Anti-Miasmatic Remedies. This concept is nothing but a Designer Genetic Medicine, which the world has not recognized yet.

9. Homeopathic doctors have done incredible work globally but still extensive research work as per the standardized methods is the need of an hour.

Chapter 4

Plant Remedies

1. Aconitum Lycoctonum

Family: Ranunculaceae; C.N. Leopard's Bane, Monkshood

This is called the first poison of the world and one of the deadliest plant.

It has been used as an arrow poison to kill wild animals like wolves and panthers; so it is named as wolf's bane.

The main causes of death include ventricular arrhythmia and asystole, or paralysis of the heart or respiratory center.

It contains diterpenoid alkaloids which are found to be effective against Multi Drug Resistant cancers in vitro.[1]

The main alkaloid is lycoctonine[2] which is used as a precursor to make Taxane, a chemotherapeutic agent effective against triple negative breast cancer. It is mainly derived from another highly poisonous plant, Taxus Baccata, which is noxious and can lead to death.

It is also indicated for Hodgkin's lymphoma and mammary cancer.

Keywords: Highly poisonous; Diterpenoids; MDR Cancers; Taxane Precursor; Lymphoma; Triple Negative Breast Cancer.

Homeopathic Indications

1. Mania.

2. Ferocity.

3. Laughter.

4. Distraction.

5. Instability of ideas.

6. Dread of work.

7. Repugnance to business changeable mood.

8. Restlessness-heat during.

9. Sleepiness.

10. Desire – sweets, fruits, delicacies, cabbage.

11. Aversion - milk, fat tobacco.

12. Aggravation - pork, onion, wine.

13. Abdomen—pain, cutting; pork after—diarrhea-pork after (beef agg. - Ipecac, Kali nit. China, Zinc, Sul.).

14. Bluish, Ulcerated gums.

15. Clayey taste.

16. Cracked skin of the nose.

17. Hodgkin's Disease.

18. Itching at the vulva.

19. Fetid menstrual blood.

20. Excoriation of the bend of the thigh after the menses.

21. Viscid leucorrhoea.

22. Swelling of the cervical glands.

23. The neck seems to grow larger.

24. Swelling of the neck on one side only.

25. Swelling of the mammary glands.

2. Anantherum Muriaticum

Family: Poaceae; C.N. Cuscus Grass, Vetiver.

From this grass root, an aromatic oil is obtained which has pleasant smell, and possesses soothing, cooling and medicinal properties.

This species has a structured root system, can go 3-4 m deep in first year of growth; is highly draught tolerant, fire and frost resistant, can endure heavy grazing pressure and survive in prolonged flow of water.

This plant acts as a stimulant and have aphrodisiac properties as well. It is often observed while homeopathic proving that a stimulant substance gives picture of excessive enervation, frenzy and exalted passion.

An Aphrodisiac nature of this substance, the name 'Andropogen' and the Homeopathic proving confirms that this plant helps to increase the production of Testosterone.

Increased level of Testosterone will give rise to symptoms of excessive sexual passion and decrease in level of Estrogen which eventually will lead to **shrinkage of ovaries, sterility, atrophy of breast, increased prolactin level, continuation of milk flow in mammae.**

Estrogen also lubricates skin, protects collagen and helps in the wound healing. Defficient Estrogen secretion produces dryness, cracks, excoriation, non-healing wounds and tendency to suppuration, especially of cervix and nipples. In fact, the Materia Medica of Anantherum is full of such kind of valuable skin indications.

Recent research has proven the anticancer activity of Anantherum Muriaticum in Breast Cancer.[3]

All these symptoms together suggest its utility in Breast Cancer, in which increased levels of Testosterone, Prolactin and

Progesterone Receptors positive cancers are the confirmatory markers. The symptomatology also points towards pathology like Paget's Disease.

This remedy is full of symptoms of pain which makes it an excellent remedy for cancer pain.

Keywords: Aphrodisiac; Mental Frenzy; Increased Testosterone; Ovarian Atrophy; Dryness of Skin; Anti-Cancer; Cancer Pain.

Homeopathic Indications

1. Ulcerated cancers, inflamed lymphatic glands.
2. A state of drunkenness and intoxication.
3. Gay humor, with disposition to laugh and sing.
4. OCD; mania for doing the same thing and visiting the same places.
5. Restless, Suspicious.
6. Monomania, i.e. going out, dressing in a grotesque manner.
7. Deformed nails with hormonal imbalance.
8. Similar to Thuja
9. Dreams of falling; the rubrics include falling, high places, from; falling, high places, from: water, into.
10. Tics.
11. Disposition to masturbate.
12. Great increase of the venereal appetite.
13. The venereal appetite is increased by every attempt to satisfy it, until it drives him to onanism and madness.
14. During coitus, all his sufferings cease, only to reappear afterwards with increased severity.
15. Ungovernable jealousy.
16. Desire to lean the head against something hard and cold.
17. Vertigo in all positions, aggravated especially by motion and strong air.

18. Desire to travel.

19. Red and yellow spots on the face; as if it had been painted with vermilion.

20. Intense scaly herpes, with falling off of the eyebrows and beard.

21. Wart-like growths on eyebrows and nose.

22. Fissured, lacerated tongue, and as if cut on its edges, bloody or brick red coating.

23. Thirst in esophagus, with fits of suffocating cough; like hydrophobia

24. Morbid hunger, wakes up in night to eat, as if he had a tapeworm.

25. Burning, unquenchable thirst. Longing for aromatic drinks.

26. Stomach: Obstinate and painful eructation, especially after eating vegetables.

27. Vomiting of food and of bile, with hunger even after eating.

28. Vomiting of pure blood, as if from the rupture of a blood - vessel in the stomach.

29. Induration of breasts or tongue or uterine cervix.

30. Liver Metastasis.

31. Inflammation and swelling of the liver, as if caused by abscesses; cramps in hepatic region, with sensation as if it was full of painful tuberosities; pulsating, burning and digging pains in region of liver; sensation as of a hard tumor starting from the pylorus, extending to the liver.

32. Abscesses, boils, ulcers, fissures, indurations, tumors, tendency to suppuration, chancre like sores, warty overgrowth.

33. Neuralgia of severest order.

34. Lancinating, burning, deep-seated pains (in tumors). Pain piercing like steel arrows.

35. Formication and itching as of ants, with loss of sensibility.

36. Coffee aggravates the pains, but afterwards relieve them.

37. Strong liquors aggravate, aromatic liquors ameliorate, the pains.
38. Green leucorrhea.
39. Leucoplakia.
40. Breasts swollen, indurated with swelling of the ganglia of the chest and axilla; burning, lancinating, and gnawing pains, as if there were live animals.
41. Congestion of the breasts as from accumulation of milk.
42. Breasts are atrophied and become soft.
43. Heat and pain in the breasts, as if they had been gashed with a penknife. Inflammation and swelling.
44. Excoriation of the nipples.
45. Painful swelling which tend to suppurate, especially sub maxillary and cervical glands.
46. The chest feels as if bound in a corset, which prevents its action.
47. Phlegmonous erysipelas in the breasts, with tendency to attack the head.

3. Aristolochialis Clematitis

The plant, commonly known as snakeroot, has been used traditionally for snakebite.

Flower of this plant resembles the natural shape of birth canal. Commonly known as birthwort, this plant is used since many centuries as a remedy to assist birth, contraception and also to induce abortion, as well as a vulnerary for injuries and joint pains.

It was used as a folk remedy to lose weight owing to its property of renal stimulator, but later on, it was found to cause End Stage Renal Disease and Urothelial Cancers.

It is a proven Carcinogen with a distinct Mutagenic Signature. It alters p53 gene.[4]

Aristolochic Acid present in this plant affects secretion of Arachidonic Acid at cellular level which activates COX 2, IL 8 pathways associated with wound healing and increased secretion of Prostaglandins. Prostaglandin E2 is responsible for cervical dilatation and renal pumping.[5]

Overexpression of these signaling is found to excite Beta Estrogen Receptors present in Urinary Bladder which, in turn, produces Bladder Carcinoma and Estrogen Positive Breast Cancer.

Keywords: p53 mutation; Arachidonic Acid, Prostaglandin; COX 2-IL 8 pathway; Beta Estrogen Receptors; Bladder and Breast Cancer

Homeopathic Indications

1. DIOSCORIDES has stated of Birthwort that the powder being drunk in wine "brings away both birth and afterbirth and whatsoever a careless midwife hath left behind."

2. Hormonal imbalance. Subjects of a nervous constitution, with extreme sensitivity.

3. Tubercular conditions of the "worn-out" type.

4. Hybrid of Sepia + Pulsatilla + Arnica; Tearful depression, fear of people but not aversion, easily offended, not easily comforted like Pulsatilla but rather inconsolable and cross when in the depression, yet not actively aggravated by consolation like Sepia.

5. Prevalence of extremes of moods, namely either a marked depression or a rather forced or unreasonable exhilaration and cheerfulness, even in alternation. Also found were extreme states of extroversion or introversion in the same person.

6. Great tiredness and exhaustion or/and alternating with unusual activity and ability to perform, i.e. the manic-depressive response pattern.

7. Insatiable hunger in spite of indigestion.

8. Poor circulation and local congestion "Venous type".

9. Tendency to cold extremities and bunions.

10. Extreme chilliness not better by external heat.

11. Most of the local symptoms are better from local heat and worse from cold.

12. Headache and coryza are better from cool air and cold application. In turn, the whole patient desires and is better by cool air.

13. Better from motion similar to Rhus Tox.

14. Better from onset of any discharge; worse before menses and better with onset of menses.

15. The general aggravation is in the morning upon rising and at 2-4 a.m. [sleep, cough].

16. Sour, bitter vomiting; vomiting after sauerkraut, better after milk.

17. Diarrhea with sudden call, so that toilet is but barely reached

18. Emotional, anticipatory enteritis and colitis.

19. Tearing, sticking pains of joints, better at onset of menses or mucous bloody leucorrhoea; worse from sewing or knitting.

20. Menopausal arthroses. Legs feel heavy like lead.

21. Excessive swelling of the extremities before menses.

22. Congestion and varicosities of pregnancy.

23. Urinary tract: Irritation, inflammation, cystitis, pyelitis, polyuria; Albuminuria; Preeclampsia. Enuresis nocturne, in old females.

24. Acne worse before menses; Dry cracked skin. Weeping eczema. Poorly healing skin. Poorly healing wounds; infected wounds.

25. Blisters from rubbing shoes, rowing, garden work, horseback riding, etc. Infected blisters from marching soldiers; external injuries from rubbing.

26. Prevents infection of fresh wounds and promotes granulation. Painful contusions, burns, frozen extremities.

27. For external application, it is more superior to Calendula.

28. Produces excess of Estrogen.

29. Indicated for conditions arising after hysterectomy, use of synthetic female hormones to defer menstruation, contraception or treat sterility.

30. In routine office work, first consideration is to be given to Aristolochialis before any other remedy [unless definitely indicated] in any case of suppressed or deficient menstruation.

31. Restores menstruation, which is too weak or suppressed, even in cases of amputation of uterus. General symptoms become better as menses reappear. Amenorrhea due to confinement in prison, camps, flight or travel.

32. Abdominal cramps before menses. Heaviest dysmenorrhea.

33. Sensation of pain and hardness in left breast.

34. Sclerocystic mastitis.

35. Chest feels hard, like a breastplate.

4. Belladonna

Belladonna is another well-known remedy from Solanaceae family. The biochemical action is similar to the Solanum Mamosum.

Homeopathic Indications

1. This medicine treats Tumors of the Breast and Metastasis.

2. Throbbing Pain with redness and streaks, radiating from the nipple.

3. The breasts feel heavy, hard and red. Pain usually occurs in short attacks, causing redness of the face and eyes with fullness of the head and throbbing of carotids.

4. Loss of appetite.

5. Great thirst for cold water.

6. Spasms of stomach.

7. Empty, retching, uncontrollable vomiting.

8. Dread of Drinking.

9. Transverse colon protrudes like a pad, tender, swollen.

10. Pain is if clutched by hand, worse jar and pressure.

11. Extreme sensitiveness to touch even of bed clothes.

12. Rush of blood to head and face (DDx Amyl, Glon., Mel.).

13. Headache congestive with red face, throbbing of brain and carotids.

14. Violent delirium, disposition to bite, spit, strike and tear things, breaks into fits of laughter and gnashes the teeth, wants to bite and strike the attendant (DDx Stram.).

15. Tries to escape (DDx Hell.).

5. Bellis Perennis

C.N. Lawn Daisy: Family: Compositae (Arnica, Calendula Family)

This plant is also an invasive weed.

Bellis Perennis is rightly described by Dr Tyler for injuries by Doctrine of Analogy that these tiny flowerheads keep on blooming even after being subjected to severe trampling.

The Family Compositae is well-known for its effects on Injuries of various kinds, wound healing and anti-inflammatory properties and have widely applied for same successfully since decades by Homeopaths across the globe.

Bellis Perennis is listed in Materia Medica as one of the remedies for breast cancer after injury. Injury implies both recent and remote ones, as well as at physical and psyche level. An Injury like sensation perceived without an actual Injury also is an indication of this remedy.

This family contains glucosides, Sesquiterpenoid Lactone, and has proved to be very effective against Breast Cancer of Estrogen Negative types.[6]

Keywords: Injury; Sesquiterpenoid Lactone, Estrogen Negative Breast Cancer

Homeopathic Indications

1. First remedy for injuries to the deeper tissues, after major surgical work.

2. Results of injuries to nerves with intense soreness and intolerance of cold bathing.

3. Complaints due to cold food or drink when the body is heated, and in affections due to cold wind.

4. Breasts and uterus engorged. Varicose veins in pregnancy. DURING PREGNANCY INABILITY TO WALK.

5. Worse, **LEFT SIDE**; before storms; cold bathing; cold wind.

6. Amelioration from movement, heat, food and pressure, cold

7. Stasis" and "fag" are the principal notes of the action.

8. Carbo-fluoric types, with tendency to visceral ptosis, laxity of the ligaments, and hemorrhages.

9. Development of chronic mesenchymatous conditions which may become cancerous.

10. Keynote symptoms are endometriosis, a history of recurrent abortion, pain in lower abdomen, a flattened cervix, trauma to female organ and PID.

11. Cancer of Breast after Injury.

12. Stasis, exudation, bruises and swelling; much more than in Arnica.

13. Patient wants to lie down.

14. Burning pain over the nodule on the breast.

15. Unbearable pains that drive to distraction

16. Wakeful too early.
17. Sensation as if going to sneeze.
18. Desire company, family, forsaken feeling.
19. Cheerful during thunder and lightning.
20. Fear of impending danger.
21. Dreams of animals.
22. Pain remaining after pregnancy.
23. Fibroids.
24. Chilly.

6. Bryonia Alba

This is an aggressive, noxious Weed from Cucurbitaceae-Cucumber family.

The name comes from word "bryo" meaning to grow vigorously.

It possesses enormously large size of roots.

The juice is very bitter, nauseous and toxic; strongly purgative and laxative in action; can be fatal.

An Algerian study has found extract of Bryonia very useful in Breast Cancer and Burkitt's Lymphoma by producing apoptosis and preventing metastasis. This property is largely attributed to its flavonoids, Kaempferols, which are proven to be very beneficial against Estrogen Positive Breast Cancer.[7]

An Indian study has found extract of Bryonia causing better cytotoxic response in Breast Cancer than Vincristine and Doxorubicin.[8]

An Armenian study has stated "Clinical trials show that the Bryonia extract was effective in treating workers at the Chernobyl Nuclear reactor who suffered from vegetovascular dystonia and other accompanying illnesses as a result of that facility's well-known accident. It was also effective in preventing radiation-induced disorders and cytostatic side effects in cancer therapy without side effects."[9]

Keywords: Laxative: cathartic; Estrogen Positive Breast Cancer; Burkitt's Lymphoma; Radiation

Homeopathy Indications

1. Irritable, inclined to be vehement and angry; dark or black hair and complexion; dry, nervous, slender people; "persons accustomed to rich living, with rich blood, firm resisting flesh."

2. Ailments from chagrin, mortification, anger; violence, with chilliness and coldness.

3. Delirium: talks constantly about his business; desire to get out of bed and go along.

4. Excessive dryness of mucous membranes with scanty expectoration; great thirst.

5. Synovial swellings.

6. Vicarious menstruation.

7. Pains; stitching, tearing, worse at night;

8. Aggravated by motion, inspiration, coughing; Warm food.

9. Ameliorated by absolute rest, and lying on painful side, cold food.

10. Inflammation and swelling of the subcutaneous glands and cellular tissue, forming small, hard knots under the skin.

11. Indolent tumors, of slow growth, with slow and imperfect suppuration.

12. Mammae heavy, of a stony hardness; pale but hard; hot and painful; must support the breasts.

13. Mammae: burning.

14. Mammae: induration: caked, an early tendency to become.

7. Chimaphilla Umbellata

Family: Ericaceae (Ledum Pal, Rhododendron, Kalmia family); C.N. Rheumatism weed; 'Pipsissewa' means 'breaking into pieces' owing to its medicinal property to break renal stone into pieces.

This is a semi-parasitic plant which partially depends upon mycorrhiza fungi to draw nutrients from the other green plants.

Chimaphillin, an active constituent of this plant is found to possess strong antifungal properties.

While studying Homeopathic symptomatology and medicinal uses of this plant, it is found useful in Organic Dropsy due to kidney or liver problems; Galactorrhea in women with large size of breast; Cancer of various kinds and Diabetes Mellitus.

After studying several hundred research papers on all above topics, it could be concluded that such pathologies together can take place when the Axis of Growth Hormone secreted by Pituitary gland and Insulin like Growth Factor (IGF 1) secreted in liver and Embryonic hormone IGF 2 are affected.

The Cancer tumors themselves behave like an embryo and many embryonic pathways which are responsible for tremendous growth potential of stem cells gets abnormally activated during malignancies. These molecular pathways are anti-apoptosis and anti-tumor suppressor.

Intrauterine fetal hormone IGF 2 is found over expressed in many cancers, diabetes and obesity as well kidney and liver diseases. In fact, abnormal value of IGF 2 is an indication of poor prognosis in several cancers.

Insulin-like Growth Hormones 2 affects the Growth hormone (GH) which gives rise to obesity, breast size which larger than the body frame with increased epithelial stroma of breast tissues and comparatively smaller ducts and ultimately adenocarcinoma and triple negative breast cancer.[10]

Growth hormone disturbances activate Prolactin which results into excessive flow of milk, also in non-pregnant women and suppression of Estrogen-Progesterone which leads to suppression of menses, reduced development of ductal part of breast and rapid atrophy of breast later as a secondary action.

In a study, acromegaly (i.e. due to excessive secretion of Growth Hormone) was found strongly associated with Prolapse of Uterus and this is noted in the symptomatology of this drug.

It is also used as a rubefacient like Belladonna, and hence, presents a symptom of circumscribed redness over cheeks.

The leaves of these plant family have sharp needle-like shape or presence of sharp teeth along the edges and implying Doctrine of Signature according to Dr R. Sankaran , the sensation in this family is of sharp needle-like pains as of injury from sharp, pointed instruments with nerve pain relieved by cold application pointing towards arctic, cold climate preference of this plant.

Keywords: Growth Hormone; IGF 2; Galactorrhea in Non-Pregnant Women, Larger breast size followed by Rapid Atrophy of Breast, Amenorrhea; Visceral dropsies; Obesity; Diabetes mellitus; Prolapse of Uterus; Fungal infections; Triple Negative breast cancer

Homeopathic Indications

1. Cachectic, Scrofulous, Broken down constitutions in intemperate subjects, abdominal and renal dropsies.
2. Frequent desire to urinate, with scanty urine; Advanced stages of albuminuria.
3. Vesical tenesmus, from prolapse or retroversion of uterus

4. Inability to pass urine without standing with feet wide apart and body inclined forward.

5. Great increase of appetite, much thirst, desire to cool tongue.

6. Tongue swollen and coated white in the middle.

7. Diabetes caused by the infection of the urinary system.

8. Rapid atrophy of breasts.

9. Suppression of Menses.

10. Painful tumor of breast in young unmarried women

11. Sharp pain: in tumor and axillae.

12. Undue secrction or suppression of milk.

13. Galactorrhea in unmarried women with large breast.

14. Lump in left breast broke, leaving small, irregular ulcer with ragged, everted edges, sloughing and discharging fetid pus.

15. Cancer of breast.

16. Scirrhous tumor of right breast, about an inch in diameter, hard, but movable, nipple drawn in, a good deal of sharp pain in tumor and in axillae.

17. Every third day, constipated stool.

18. Aggravation: Cold damp; sitting on cold places: left side. Amelioration: Walking.

19. Complementary: Kali Mur.

8. Cistus Canadensis

Order: Malvales, Family: Cistaceae; C.N. Frostweed; Rock Rose.

This is thermophilus plant requiring open, sunny places. The genus of this plant is peculiar as it possess a range of specific adaptation to resist summer draught and frequent disturbance events, such as fire and grazing.

The seeds grow after getting heated by wildfire (similar to effects of Radiation).

Various Cistus *species are known to emit volatile oils, rendering the plants flammable. Some sources* have stated that under dry, hot conditions, these species may be capable of self-ignition.

It is one of the known Bach Flower Remedies used to treat conditions arising after Horror, Terror and Emergency.

After studying the phytochemistry of Rockrose, the extreme Sensitiveness to Cold can be explained to Thermophilus nature of this plant, but there is no carcinogenic element is obtained. The homeopathic proving confirms its use for indurated neck glands and Breast Tumors.

But rhizomes of this plant share a symbiotic relationship with Agaricales group of edible mushroom of Boletus and Laccata Species. These fungi are rich sources of Mercury and are documented for their anticancer properties. In fact, they are considered to be one of the most promising anticancer drugs.

The Agaricales species is known to inhibit Aromatase Enzyme. This is associated with Estrogen Positive Breast Cancer in Postmenopausal women.[11]

Aromatase enzyme activity is found to be affected by temperature in primates which also correlates with extreme thermosensitive nature of Cistus Patients.

Keywords: Thermosensitivity; History of unresolved emotions of Horror, Terror and Fright; Agaricus + Mercury; Aromatase Inhibition; Estrogen Positive Breast Cancer in Post-Menopausal Women; Radiation

Homeopathic Indications

1. Flabby, pale, sickly persons who cannot ascend the stairs without losing their breath.
2. Extreme sensitivity to cold; very chilly.

3. Hemorrhagic Cancers.

4. Neurological Lesions.

5. Twitching; Extremities. Involuntary drawing and trembling feeling in the muscular parts of the hands and lower extremities, with pain in the wrists, fingers, and knee joints.

6. A bruised pain in all the limbs, as from fatigue; great sensitiveness to touch, worse from touch.

7. Sensation as if ants were running through the whole bed.

8. Loquacity.

9. Sensation of coldness of tongue, larynx and trachea.

10. Saliva cool, breath feels cool.

11. Desire for acid food and fruits.

12. Scorbutic, swollen gums, separating from teeth, easily bleeding, putrid, disgusting.

13. Cancer of the breast, pharynx, or neck and gives rise to very marked cervical adenopathy; the glands of the neck enlarge like ropes in lines.

14. Stitches in the throat, causing cough, whenever mentally agitated.

15. "Spongy" feeling in the throat; Continuous feeling of dryness and heat in the throat. Must get up in the night, on account of dryness in the throat. In the night, swallowing of saliva, on account of dryness. After eating or drinking, the dryness is relieved; < after sleeping causing Insomnia (Note: such kind symptoms are frequently caused due to Radiation Therapy and the vary behavior of these plant suggest it to be the remedy for the effects of Radiation and Burns).

16. Cancer of mammae with amenorrhea.

17. Asthma > by fresh air.

9. Clematis Erecta

Family Ranunculaceae, Pulsatilla - Stayphisagria family; C.N. 'Pepper Vine'.

Acrid leaves are used as a pepper substitute. Merely touching the leaves of this plant can raise blisters, n this is due to presence of Protoanemonin which gives a very good anti-inflammatory and analgesic properties.

Clematis erecta is an aggressive weedy plant with proliferative growth and capacity to smother any plant which comes in between. It is a vine which can equally grow covering the ground and such growth potential is attributed to its capacity to resist microbes and plant parasites.

Numerous scientific researchers have established Clematis as an excellent antifungal/yeast medicine, useful especially against Candida and a superlative antibacterial of gram positive and negative strains including Neisseria gonorrhea.[12]

These are not just simple superficial skin infections, but quite deeper, chronic infections involving many systems and organs giving rise to multiple pathologies. Chronic Yeast and Staphylococcus infection may pass through breast milk giving rise to mastitis and oral thrush. Such chronic inflammatory conditions make the individual prone to Cancer.

Invasive candidiasis, especially of genitourinary organ, produces a lipid metabolite which mimics Prostaglandin, thus overactivating COX 2 pathway, which, in turn, produces urothelial pathologies like stricture, carcinoma, uterine pathologies and ultimately Estrogen positive Breast Cancer.[13]

Clematis works quite similarly to Aristolochialis Clematitis in its action, but history of chronic Candida/Yeast and chronic bacterial infection will be differentiating point.

The peppery, acrid nature provoked on mere touching, can be related to oversensitive nature of Pulsatilla, Staphysagria along with angry, irritable temperament of mind and physical complaints.

Keywords: Touchy-Edgy nerves; Protoanemonin; Antifungal; Antibacterial; Chronic Infections; Candidiasis, Prostaglandin E; COX 2 Pathway; Estrogen Positive Breast Cancer

Homeopathic Indications

1. Acts best on light-haired people, torpid, cachectic conditions, swellings and indurations of the glandular system, syphilitic taint.

2. Pulsatilla-like mind symptoms along with urinary complaints.

3. Mind similar to Sepia, for disgusting, hitting children.

4. Fear of being alone but disinclined to meet otherwise agreeable company.

5. Effects of homesickness, with restless, dreamy sleep and vibratory sensations throughout the body.

6. Pulsations felt throughout the body.

7. Clinical Keynote is commencing stricture.

8. Sleepiness.

9. > Perspiration.

10. < Moon.

11. Rheumatism.

12. Inability to pass all the urine, dribbling after urinating.

13. Tobacco Toothache.

14. Ringworm with intolerable itching in bed and after washing; eruptions following suppressed gonorrhea; eruptions moist during increasing and dry during decreasing moon.

15. Deep ulcers; indurated ulcers, with high, elevated edges, serous, yellow, acrid and ichorous; scanty secretion or total suppression of pus.

16. Menses: premature.
17. Scirrhous mammae, with stitches in shoulder and gland, very painful during increasing moon.
18. MAMMAE: CANCER: SCIRRHUS: LEFT, OF, VERY PAINFUL, WORSE IN COLD WEATHER AND DURING NIGHT, WORSE DURING GROWING MOON, WHILE PERSPIRING SHE CANNOT BEAR TO BE UNCOVERED.
19. MAMMAE: INDURATION: GLANDULAR, ABOUT NIPPLE, PAINFUL TO TOUCH.

10. Condurango

Family: Apocynaceae, Milkweed, the cut latex of this plant oozes milk and weedy in nature so the name Milkweed; other well-known remedies of the same family include Indian drugs like Calotropis and G. Sylvester; the milk from cut latex is used to remove warts topically.

Parts used: The bark of the plant is used.

It belongs to Vinca Minora family from which a chemotherapeutic drug Vincristine is obtained.

Current researchers attribute the therapeutic potential of milkweed family to fungal endophytes present in the bark of these plants which are responsible for the biogenesis of various plant alkaloids.

A very strong characteristic of this remedy is angular stomatitis and according to pathology which is due to fungal infection, Candidiasis.

From homeopathic proving, it is inferred that this drug possess strong antifungal properties.

In fact, the active alkaloid, Conduritol, is a cyclohexene kind of carcinogen; an established Beta Glucosidase inhibitor and proven to be effective against chronic fungal/ infection and various kind of Cancers, especially multi-drug resistant cancer.

Glucosidase inhibitors are of great use in the treatment of MDR infections of Gastrointestinal Tract, Diabetes and Lysosomal storage diseases.[14]

Chronic Candidiasis makes one prone to malignancy giving rise to Estrogen positive Breast Cancer through the action on COX 2 pathway (DDX Clematis Erecta). Clematis has more affinity for genitourinary tract while Condurango seems to have for Gastrointestinal tract.

Keywords: Angular Stomatitis; Conduritol; Glucosidase Inhibitor; Candidiasis; Gastritis; Diabetes Mellitus, Lysosomal Storage Disease; MDR Estrogen Positive Breast Cancer

Homeopathic Indications

1. Cracks along the Muco-cutaneous Junction (Nit Acid, Nat Mur but Cond. lacks the stabbing pain).
2. Mouth Commissures; Ulcerated.
3. Tongue unusually Clear and Red.
4. Locomotor Ataxia; Staggering Gait.
5. Weakness of Lower Limbs.
6. Complete loss of appetite, emaciation.
7. Unclean Ulcers with surrounding hardness and swelling.
8. Feeling of soreness, like rheumatism, through the left shoulder and under the left scapula.
9. Tendency to metastasis to Liver, Esophagus, Stomach and Intestine.
10. Organic stenosis of esophagus.
11. A contraction localized under the umbilical, right or left.
12. Cancers originating in the epithelial tissues; excrescences are strong indications for its use.
13. MAMMAE: CANCER: SCIRRHUS: DISCHARGE, ULCERATION WITH FETID SANIOUS, AND SLOUGHING.

14. MAMMAE: CANCER: SCIRRHUS: PURPLE, SKIN, IN SPOTS AND WRINKLED

15. MAMMAE: CANCER: SCIRRHUS: SKIN AND AXILLARY GLANDS INVOLVED

16. MAMMAE: TUMORS: HARD, VERY, INCOMPRESSIBLE. KNOBBY, IMMOVABLE, LANCINATING PAINS.

17. NIPPLES: RETRACTED: SCIRRHUS.

18. One of the best remedies to relieve the stinging, burning pains of Cancer.

11. Conium Maculatum

This is the toxic weed from Umbelliferae family, C.N. Poison Hemlock. Conium word comes from 'Konas' means to whirl around from the symptom of vertigo felt after ingesting this plant.

It is the famous "Poison Hemlock" which was given to Socrates to drink to die. Conium produces ascending type of paralysis till the respiratory, cardiac muscle fail to death.

It is teratogenic by nature. Cattle who used to graze this plant gave birth to babies with Congenital Malformations like cleft palate, multiple congenital contractures, etc.

Most of the anti-cancer drugs are teratogenic in nature. Cancer cells behave like an embryo and the intrauterine neural pathways, which generally gets deactivated after the birth, gets reactivated during malignancy. They are responsible for uncontrolled growth of malignant cells. Teratogens work over these pathways and block them. Anti-cancer drugs and teratogens act like two sides of the same coin.

Conium has a toxic alkaloid, Coniine, which is similar to Nicotine in action. It works on the Nicotine Acetylcholine Receptors of the Nervous system.

These receptors are responsible for transmission of messages at the Synapse of Neuromuscular Junction, therefore it produces paralysis and muscle contracture.

Excessive and abnormal stimulation of nACh Receptors by Nicotine through consumption of tobacco products, also stimulates Estrogen receptors in brain, and as a consequence leads to hormone positive Breast Cancer.[15]

Conium works on the same neural pathway and produces and cures malignancy, especially when there is a history of Tobacco abuse.

In olden times, the juice of Conium was applied on the breast of young nuns to arrest their sexual development.

One of well-known indication of Conium is malignancy caused due to prolonged suppression of sexual desire or Celibacy. Such suppression of natural instinct leads to excessive prolactin level in the system, which leads to decreased Estrogen levels, shrinkage of mammary glands and suppression of menses. This can be confirmed by increased prolactin level in the blood.

Being the member of Umbelliferae family, it shares common symptoms of intolerance to light; band or hoop like sensation around parts; terrors at mental level and stabbing, knife-like pains.

Keywords: Teratogen; Coniine; Vertigo; Nicotine Receptors; Synapses; Paralysis; Celibacy, Increased Prolactin; Estrogen Positive Breast Cancer

Homeopathic Indications

1. Depressed, timid, averse to society, yet fears being alone.
2. No inclination for business or study. Indifferent. Difficulty in understanding what he is reading. Superstitious. Unable to sustain mental effort.

3. Thinks that animals are jumping on his bed. Sad; dissatisfied with herself and Surroundings. Cannot think after using eyes.
4. Cares very little for things; makes useless purchases, wastes or ruins them. Likes to wear his best clothes.
5. Sadness worse by sympathy. As if great guilt weighed upon him. Fears when alone, but dread of strangers or company, during menses.
6. Vertigo aggravated by turning head, turning sideways, seeing moving objects; ameliorated by closing eyes.
7. Perspiration Sleep During, even while closing the eyes.
8. Perspiration Under Eyes.
9. Intense photophobia.
10. Earwax blood red.
11. Constant desire to swallow from a lump in the throat. Food goes the wrong way when swallowing.
12. Coldness of stool and flatus.
13. Flatulence from Milk.
14. Debility (old age, over - indulgence) or paralysis spreads from below upward. Lower part of the body gives way before the upper. Weakness of legs; tottering gait. Numbness of all parts with weakness and cold feet.
15. Painlessness.
    a. *Aggravation: during eating, while standing, while lying down (cough), while at rest, when lifting the affected part, from masturbation.*
    b. *Amelioration: in the dark; from letting the affected limb hang down, from moving, when walking*
16. Cancerous tumors in old, unmarried females or those whose sexual life was suddenly withdrawn.
17. Cancer of the Breast after bruises or injuries.
18. Hypertrophy of breast, either general or lobular, followed by wasting of breasts, complete atrophy of mammary gland, leaving a flaccid, bag like skin.

19. Severe stitches, like knife thrusts, in the side, with loud cries on this account. Violent stitches in the right side of the chest about the nipple, on every inspiration while walking, relieved by hard pressure with the hand.

20. Tumor in the breast of size of walnut, tea cup, hen's egg, uneven of stony hardness; the mass is immovable, and skin covering it not discolored.

21. Concealed Cancer of bones; Caries of sternum.

22. Bleeding of ulcers with a secretion of fetid ichor.

23. Ovarian depression with amenorrhea; atrophy of ovaries with sterility.

24. TUMORS: clavicular fossa.

25. FLABBY MAMMAE: MENSES, EXCEPT DURING.

26. Milk: thin: watery, and: long after weaning.

27. INNER   CHEST: TENSION: PAINFUL,   WITH HEMORRHAGE   OR   HEMOPTYSIS,   ESPECIALLY AFTER MASTURBATION.

28. VOICE: HOARSE: LEUCORRHOEA, AFTER.

29. RETRACTION of nipples.

30. INDURATION: Mammae: hard, very: hard as stones: parturition, after.

31. CANCER: Mammae: menses, during absence of.

32. INDURATION: Mammae: bunch, in.

The symptoms and study of this plant phytochemistry indicates Conium to be remedy for Estrogen positive Breast Cancer with increased Prolactin level, of either side, origin being from Uterus or Ovaries. Tendency for growth and metastasize to axilla, clavicle along with multiple metastasis including lungs, stomach and bones. The strong family history of cancer and tobacco consumption is noted in this remedy. Also, it can be used for epithelial or Paget's disease like pathology.

12. Galium Aparine

Family: Rubiaceae (China, Ipecac, Coffee family).

C.N.: Cleavers, Goose Grass; **Weedy** and **invasive plant**, has got hairy root like structures which clings to fur of an **animal** passing nearby to get **dispersed**.

It is used as a cheaper substitute for coffee with less caffeine and a tonic to lose weight. It is also used as cleanser and for lymphatic drainage. Used as a poultice for injury, burns, cancerous ulcers and stings of venomous insects.

It is used since many years as a remedy for gravel and kidney tonic, fever as well for cancer.

Cleaver is used as a natural red color dye like its close relative Madder, Rubbia Tinctoria. The red pigment is due to presence of anthraquinone alkaloid, which closely resembles anthracycline group of drugs (a red pigmented compound isolated from Streptomyces P. bacteria and precursor of **Rubidomycin** chemotherapeutic drug).

From this, **Doxorubicin**, one of the leading chemotherapeutic agents, is formulated which is cytotoxic, myelosuppressive and cardiotoxic drug.

Doxorubicin is used for triple negative and aggressive type of breast cancer as well for leukemia and lymphoma. Gallium Aparine is also found useful for the **Triple Negative type of Breast Cancer**

Current researchers have confirmed the effect of Gallium Aparine as a cytotoxic and anti-apoptotic drug and suggest its use as an anticancer drug.

It is found to act through the cancer causing **ERK-MAPK pathway.**[17]

The presence of Caffeine in Gallium gives it an excessive nervine stimulation like Coffea, also giving bitter taste as well as a painkilling and sedative effect.

Keywords: Doxorubicin; Erk-Mapk Pathway; Triple Negative Breast Cancer; Caffeine

Homeopathic Indications

1. Inveterate skin affections and scurvy.
2. Urinary Lithiasis.
3. Patients with multiple neurofibroma.
4. Epithelioma, slow in its progress, having nodular deposits around the surface.
5. Favors healthy granulations over ulcerated surfaces.
6. Nodulated tumor on tongue.
7. Has power of suspending or modifying cancerous affection.
8. After surgery, primary lesion metastasizes to faraway places.
9. Affinity for Liver, Blood metastasis.

13. Hoang Nan

Family: Loganiaceae (Nux Vomica- Ignatia family); C.N.: Tropical Bindweed,.

This plant has stems which twist and grow over other plants, prolific leaves shun out the sunlight causing them to die by starving.

It has deep roots, nearby dispersed seeds remain viable for many years, and vegetative buds are capable of arising along a lateral root.

It smothers everything in the path, and one cannot get rid of it. If one pulls it, it breaks but only to come back with vengeance, bigger and stronger than ever. Brush killer or pesticides are of no use to stop the growth of the prolific plant.

Like other members of this family, this plant contains Strychnine and Brucine.

Both these alkaloids work over Nicotine Acetyl Choline Receptors and Glycine receptors as antagonists, and this way affects the neuromuscular junctions causing excessive startling, hyper reflexes, convulsions, tonic and clonic spasms, breakdown of musculature and paralysis as a secondary action. Primary action is observed mainly over the brain and the spinal cord.

Overstimulation of both these receptors, especially Nicotine one, is strongly associated with altered neurotransmitters, stress hormones, endothelial growth factors and ultimately to tobacco and trauma/stress related malignancies. This also affects the nerve endings, either making them oversensitive to pain, making them numb as a secondary action similar to paralysis.

These molecular pathways are associated with genesis of Estrogen positive Breast Cancer, not responding to hormone therapy, spreading to lung, liver or brain. (DDX Conium)

Mechanism of action of this drug is quite similar to Conium, and both share paralytic affection with cancer of glandular structure and history of abuse of tobacco.

But overstimulation of these pathways arise from a sudden shock due to fear and fright leading to disturbances of sex hormones in Conium while in Hoang nan the trauma is due to shock from a shattering loss as if experienced due to sudden death (like Ignatia) in close family leading to stress hormones like adrenalin and cortisol in an attempt to cope with a stress of loss.

The phytochemistry study of these plant also reveals them to be very good medicines for Glioma.

The invasive, weedy nature of Hoang Nan makes it a superior choice for Cancer when symptoms of Ignatia are present and there is strong history of emotional trauma/grief associated with malignancy, or when there is excessive indulgence in tobacco/ drug abuse as a coping mechanism for stress like Nux Vomica.

Keywords: Synapses-Brain-Spinal Cord; Nicotine Receptors; Sudden Trauma and prolonged stress; Hyperreflexia and Paralysis; Numbness, Estrogen Resistant Breast Cancer

Homeopathic Indications

1. Bleeding Cancers.
2. Offensiveness.
3. Related to Arsenic Album.
4. Hypoesthesia of skin.
5. H/O of snake bite, hydrophobia.
6. Fatigue, general indisposition, vertigo, tingling of the hands and feet, involuntary movements of jaw.
7. Mental lassitude, indisposition to effort.
8. Malignant ulcers, pustular eczema, boils, carbuncles, leprosy.
9. Constipation alternating with diarrhea.
10. Cancer: Epithelioma.

14. Hydrastis Canadensis

Family: Ranunculaceae; C.N.: Golden seal; Parts used: Rhizome.

It was used as plant dye for yellow color. It is often observed while studying cancer remedies that either they are invasive weeds by biological nature, often a substance used as a dye for coloring or both.

This is native American Plant Remedy used as an herbal wash for antibacterial/fungal/viral purposes, similar to Indian Curcumin. It is very popular and widely used for its different medicinal virtues that its almost on the verge of extinction and declared as an endangered plant species.

This is one of very popular cancer remedies and also claimed as a carcinogenic in a study at Canada. According to the principle of Homeopathy, if it can produce cancer, it will cure cancer.

It contains alkaloids, Hydrastine and Berberine, which are cytotoxic in vivo and vitro.

If taken in large doses, it produces a train of symptoms including oversecretion of mucous membranes. If persisted, it produces severe ulceration of any surface it may touch; and catarrhal inflammation followed by extreme dryness and fission. It also causes severe inflammation of the mucous lining of the Gall Bladder and Hepatic Ducts with icteric hue of skin and a similar condition of bladder causing catarrhal cystitis.

It proves "Doctrine of Signature" as a reliable guide to have a soft clue to medicinal property. It is found to be useful against Staphylococcus Aureus Infection (inflammatory product is often of golden yellow color) via affecting Efflux pump as well as for Liver Cancer (Bile=Yellow).[18]

It is also indicated for Breast Cancer and is found used to act in a similar manner to its sister Clematis erecta, from same botanical family. While Clematis action is centered around Genitourinary System, Hydrastis targets Hepatobiliary system.

It is indicated for chronic bacterial and fungal infections as it acts via Prostaglandin and COX 2 pathways, thus can treat Estrogen Positive Breast Cancer.

Hydrastis Muriaticum, chloride salt of alkaloid Hydrastis, is advocated for bleeding malignant ulcers of uterus, lungs, mouth, etc. with a history of fibroid uterus as well as an external application for cancer treatment when Hydrastis is indicated and given internally.

On emotional sphere, morbid sensitivity of the Ranunculaceae gets manifested giving a picture similar to Staphysagria /Pulsatilla with melancholia, as seen with most of the remedies affecting liver. At the physical level, there will be hypersensitive nerves and non-healing, painful ulcers akin to acridity of the plant juice, which altogether makes it a remedy for various cancer pains.

Keywords: Yellow; Staphylococcus Aureus; Liver and Gall Bladder, COX 2 Pathway, Estrogen Positive Breast Cancer

Homeopathic Indication

1. Cachexia.
2. Gastritis.
3. Constipation.
4. Progressive Debility with viscid, yellow, ropy discharge.
5. Wasting Emaciation.
6. EXCITEMENT: CURSES HIS MOTHER, THROWS FOOD OR MEDICINE ACROSS ROOM.
7. TALKING: AVERSE TO: MARASMUS, IN GENERAL.
8. Cancer and cancerous state, before ulceration; when pain is the principal symptom.
9. Started During Puberty or Pregnancy.
10. Desire to snub who differed.
11. Hyperthyroidism and Goiter.
12. Cancer of Breast, Nipple Retracted; Sore; Cracked in Nursing Women.
13. Cancer Mammae: With Cracks in Corners of Mouth (Condu.; Clematis Erecta).
14. Right Sided Carcinoma of Breast.
15. Tumor Hard, Adherent; Skin, mottled, puckered.
16. Cancer Mammae; Old Cicatrices.
17. Pain in Breast on Sneezing.

18. <by inspiration of cold air in dry weather, in open air and in a room with open windows, by slight discharge of blood.

19. MAMMAE: ENLARGEMENT: HARD, IRREGULAR.

20. MAMMAE: LANCINATING: LIKE KNIVES THRUST INTO.

21. MAMMAE: LANCINATING: SHOULDER, TO, AND DOWN ARMS.

22. MAMMAE: PAIN: APPEARANCE, WORN AND HAGGARD.

23. MAMMAE: PAIN: LEFT, IN, PREVENTS REST AT NIGHT.

24. MAMMAE: TUMORS: HARD, STONY, NODULATED, NOT ATTACHED TO SKIN, MOVABLE AND AS LARGE AS A FILBERT, LANCINATING PAINS.

25. UTERUS: DISCHARGE: HOT WATER, OF, WETS BED AND CLOTHES.

26. Desire for Coition during albuminous leucorrhoea with pain; while extreme aversion to coition when leucorrhoea ceases.

15. Lapsana Communis

One more medicine worth mentioning and considering for the similar conditions is **Lapsana Communis**, also known as **Nipplewort** as the closed buds of the flowers resemble human breast nipple; belong to Compositae family.

It is also an invasive weed and known as a folk medicine for chapped nipples, breast ulcers, mastitis and weaning of breast milk.

Its weedy nature, anti-cancer potential and Doctrine of Signature suggests it to be of service for breast cancer; still it requires clinical and scientific confirmation.

16. Lobelia Erinus

Family: Campanulaceae; C.N.: Asthma weed; Puke weed.

The plant is known for intensely colored, profuse bloom of flowers it produces.

The leaves are bitter in taste and produces profuse salivation. It is called asthma weed and used as a herbal expectorant in many respiratory conditions like bronchitis, asthma and whooping cough.

It can induce vomiting and employed for the same purpose, hence called puke weed.

This plant is also called 'Indian Tobacco' due to its striking similarities with Tobacco constituents.

It is used as an herbal substitute of Tobacco for de-addiction.

The active piperidine alkaloid, Lobeline, is quite similar to Nicotine in action. It binds with Nicotine Acetyl Choline Receptors at neuromuscular junction (DDX Conium, Hoang Nan) and alters dopamine secretion which enables it to regulate addictive tendencies too. Effect over nACh Receptors explains how it can be employed in the treatment of paralysis and estrogen positive breast cancer.[19] (Refer Conium for more details)

Lobeline is found useful to treat the sensitivity of Multi-Drug Resistant Breast Cancer and other cancers.[20]

Keywords: Expectorant; Tobacco Deaddiction; N Ach Receptors; Dopamine; Estrogen Positive Breast Cancer

Homeopathic Indications

1. Low spirits, dyspnoea, and flatulence.
2. Great depression following heat and perspiration.
3. MALIGNANT GROWTHS, extremely rapid development.

4. Distaste for brandy.
5. Cork-screw-like pains in abdomen.
6. Great dryness of skin, nasal and buccal mucous membranes.
7. Dry, eczematous patches covering points of first fingers.
8. Epithelioma.
9. Keratitis, interstitial.
10. Deafness with history of otorrhea, anaemia.
11. Deafness of both ears, dating from excision of tonsils at seven years old, and rapidly getting worse.
12. Menses come on too often, with much bearing down last time, this bearing down kept on for a month, being worse at the period.
13. Axillary tenderness and a large, soft swelling.
14. Right breast eaten away by cancer, "heavenly relief to local pain and distress.
15. Left breast indurated and discharging. Left breast with scattered indurated nodules over adjacent tissues, burning and stinging pains, left arm swollen.

17. Ornithogalum Umbellatum

Family Liliaceae, C.N.: Star of Bethlehem.

It is an aggressive invasive spreader, resistant to herbicides, the only way to stop its spread is to painstakingly dig up all the bulbs.

A Bach flower remedy associated with unresolved emotional trauma, shock and their after-effects.

It is found to contain Cardiac Glycoside, **Convallotoxin,**[21] which affects the Adrenaline Receptors; Sodium pump and found to be useful in the treatment of Cardiac Failure, Angina Pectoris and various types of Cancer via altering multiple pathways chiefly $Na^+K^+ATPase$ and altering ROS **(Reactive oxygen species)** leading to Carcinogenesis.

Chronic stress due to unresolved mental/emotional trauma leads to excess adrenaline secretion, increased heart rates, hypertension and tumorigeneses.

This action is quite similar to Sanguinaria Canadensis from Opium Family.

In a research, Convallotoxin was found to show anticytotoxic effects against Triple Negative Breast Cancer than Hormone positive ones.[22]

Liliaceae family acts against sphincters of the body and this remedy also acts against esophageal and gastric cancers.

Keywords: Convallotoxin; History of Emotional trauma, Sodium Pump; Hypertension, Cardiac arrythmias, Gastritis; Triple Negative Breast Cancer

Homeopathic Indications

1. Breast Cancer + Stomach Cancer.
2. < cold drinks.
3. > by warm food.
4. Tongue red and coated at back.
5. Gets cold before the pains.
6. Depression of spirits. Complete prostration. Feeling of sickness keeps patient awake at night.
7. Restlessness on account of creepy feeling in feet, cannot sit still, cannot read without walking about.
8. Feels a pressure in every nerve of the body.
9. Gastric ulceration even with hemorrhage. PAINS INCREASED WHEN FOOD PASSES PYLORIC OUTLET. VOMITING OF COFFEE-GROUND LOOKING MATTER.
10. FLATULENCE, swollen feeling across lower chest; whenever she turns in bed, FEELS AS IF A BAG OF WATER also turned inside abdomen.

11. Agonizing feeling in chest and stomach, starting from the pylorus with a flatus that rolls in balls from one side to the other, loss of appetite, phlegmy retching, and loss of flesh.

18. Phellandrium Aquaticum

Phellandrium is another remedy from Umbelliferae Family of Conium. It is also a neurotoxic remedy producing convulsions, paralysis and death, if consumed, especially the tuberous roots.

But unlike Conium, it is an aquatic plant and possesses a wine like pleasant fragrance attributed to presence of a volatile oil, Phellandrene, which is also an active constituent of Eucalyptus.

This essential oil works well on respiratory system and found to be useful against lung cancer, breast cancer lines and leukemia in vitro.[16]

Like Conium, it is also found to bind with Nicotine Receptors.

Its Homeopathic symptomatology portrays rich lung symptoms along with affinity for breast ducts and nipples.

From this, it can be concluded that it is an indicated remedy for Breast Cancer involving ducts and nipples with a tendency to metastasis to lungs.

Homeopathic Indications

1. The symptoms show a general resemblance to those of the poisonous Umbeliferaea vertigo, headache, nausea, vomiting, diarrhea, drowsiness and weakness.
2. Phelland. is suited to: Persons of a feeble, irritable, lymphatic temperament, with weak and deficient nutrition.
3. Peevish arrogance.
4. EVERYTHING TASTES SWEET.

5. Offensive eructation, smelling of bed-bugs.

6. "Desire for acids."

7. Sexual Organs: Menstruation flowing only morning and evening.

8. Headache; involving nerves going to eye.

9. Abnormal sleepiness following confinement.

10. "Universal Cough Remedy."

11. A very good remedy for the OFFENSIVE EXPECTORATION AND COUGH IN PHTHISIS, bronchitis, and emphysema. Tuberculosis, affecting generally the middle lobes.

12. Worse during growing moon.

13. < when quietly seated, standing, or lying down, >movement and in open air.

14. Intolerance of light and sound; ameliorated by eating (Lith., Psor.).

15. Deterioration of mother's health from nursing.

16. The proving developed many symptoms in both mammae, especially the right, stitches shooting inward, up to sacrum; being most marked.

17. The keynote is "Intolerable pain in lactiferous tubes between the acts of nursing." "Pain in nipples on each application of child." Either breast may be affected, but the right breast and nipple were more affected than the left; the pain appearing after nipples were healed.

18. Chest: Sharp stitches extending inward beneath the left mamma, not affected by breathing. Very violent stitches extend through the whole left mammae.

19. MAMMAE: PAIN: RIGHT, CAUSING PHYSICAL AND MENTAL DISTRESS, SO THAT SHE LOST HER STRENGTH, AND WAS SEIZED WITH SPELLS OF HYSTERICAL WEEPING.

19. Phytolacca Decandra

Poke Weed, another invasive weed, has got succulent roots and a central taproot which grows deep, spreading horizontally; survives fire due to its ability to sprout from the roots again.

Its purple juice of berries was previously used as a dye. It is poisonous in nature and can be lethal.

The OARDC staff scientists has noted that immediate and subsequent symptoms of poisoning from pokeweed include "a burning sensation in the mouth, salivation, gastrointestinal cramps, and vomiting and bloody diarrhea". Depending upon the amount consumed, more severe symptoms can occur, including "anaemia, altered heart rate and respiration, convulsions and death from respiratory failure."

It is used by herbal doctors as a medicine to treat joint, kidney, lung and skin problems.

Recently, scientists has also found various compounds of therapeutic interest from this plant. Amongst them, one is "Pokeweed Mitogen" which is found to proliferate lymphocytes, especially T-lymphocytes and other Antiviral and Antifungal Proteins which inactivates RNA, increases CD4, CD8, CD12 and CD19 counts.

These compounds are very potent cytotoxic and immunomodulatory in nature.[23]

These findings indicate Phytolacca to be the medicine for Leukemia/Lymphoma/Sarcoma; Immunodeficiency diseases like HIV and other autoimmune diseases.

Phytolacca is found effective against breast cancer in both crude and homeopathic preparations. Its immunomodulatory profile makes it a candidate for Inflammatory and Triple negative kind of Aggressive Breast Cancer/lymphoma/sarcoma which are highly metastatic in nature .

In homoeopathy, Phytolacca berries are known to reduce obesity by acting on adipose tissues in their crude form and this characteristic makes it a candidate for cachexia and weight loss related to Cancer and other autoimmune diseases.

Keywords: Pokeweed Mitogen; T Cell Lymphocyte; Antiviral; Antifungal; CD4-CD8-CD12-CD19; HIV; Triple Negative Breast Cancer

Homeopathic Indications

1. Causation; emotion, grief, bathing, injuries, blows etc., exposure to cold damp weather.
2. It stands in between Rhus Tox and Bryonia.
3. Pain Flying like Electric Shocks; shooting, lancinating, rapidly shifting; worse from motion and night.
4. Behaves like Hyoscyamus; Exhibitionist; Shameless.
5. Right - sided pains and complaints.
6. Night<; Syphilitic Background.
7. Profuse Perspiration.
8. Cannot drink hot liquids.
9. Slowly Spreading Ulcer.
10. Purple Hue of Breast Skin; very hard and sensitive mammae.
11. When Child Nurses, pain goes from nipples to all over the body.
12. Cracks and small ulcer about nipples.
13. Galactorrhea.
14. Watery, Bloody Discharge from Nipple.
15. Irritable and nervous; cannot endure pain, it is intolerable; burning pains in the ulcerations of cancer.
16. Hardness apparent from the start, caked breast, gathered breast, with large, fistulous, gaping and angry ulcers.

17. LEUCORRHEA: PROFUSE: NABOTHIAN GLANDS SWOLLEN, THICK, TENACIOUS, IN WOMEN WHO HAVE SUFFERED FROM INFLAMED OR BROKEN BREASTS AND VARIOUS GLANDULAR SWELLINGS OR ABSCESSES.

18. MENSES: DURING: SECRETIONS, INCREASE OF TEARS, SALIVA, BILE AND URINE.

19. MAMMAE: CANCER: HEN'S EGG IN, SIZE OF.

20. MAMMAE: ENLARGEMENT: HYPERTROPHY.

21. MAMMAE: INDURATION: NODOSITIES: NODULATED, ACUMINATED APPEARANCE OF NODULES.

22. MAMMAE: TUMORS: PAIN EXTENDING DOWN ARMS. (0>1>0)

23. MAMMAE: ULCERS: FISTULOUS.

24. Habitual costiveness; continual inclination to stool, but often passes only fetid flatus.

25. Modalities; aggravated by damp weather; night; ameliorated by lying down; open air.

20. Sanguinaria Canadensis

Family: Papaveraceae (Opium Family), C.N. "Blood Root."

It stores sap in the rhizomes **that grows shallowly under soil surface** over many years, the branching rhizomes can grow into a large colony.

Its juice is very acrid and kills animal cells by blocking Na^+ and K^+ transmembrane proteins, and applying the juice on skin causes tissue to die and **slough off**. It was previously used in toothpaste to remove plaque but the side effects caused **premalignant condition called Leukoplakia.** It is also used by herbal practitioners since years as an external application in Cancer Salves.

It contains **Benzyl quinoline alkaloids.**

Recent research on phytochemistry has confirmed its use as one of the gem herbs for various kinds of cancer.[24]

It is found to work on the Adrenal Receptors causing Vasoconstriction leading to determination of blood flow, conditions like Hypertension, Cardiovascular accidents due to platelet aggregation, altering the Sodium-Potassium transmembrane potential.

This change leads to alter the redox reactions at intracellular level giving rise to altered Reactive Oxygen Species production.

Altered ROS leads to damage to DNA, alter many cellular pathways leading to Carcinogenesis.

In another research, it was also found to activate **Human Myeloid Cells,** associated with **Basal like Breast Cancer out of the Duct metastasizing to the bones.**[25]

Keywords: Acridity;   Adrenal   Receptors;   Vasomotor Constrictions; ROS; Basal Like Breast Cancer

Homeopathic indications

1. "Hopefulness" of mind like in Tuberculinum.
2. Right sided remedy.
3. Vasomotor constriction.
4. Circumscribed Redness.
5. Hypertension.
6. Sleeps with eyes open.
7. Palpitation.
8. Hot flushes.
9. Menopause.
10. Periodicity.
11. Severe kind of pains, Burning like hot water.

12. Burning of palms and soles; compelled to throw off bedclothes; painful enlargement of breasts; when Lachesis and Sulphur fail to relieve.

13. Eruption on face of young women, especially during scanty menses (Bellis., Cal., Eug. j., Psor.).

14. As a dynamic remedy for the narcosis of Opium.

15. Offensive and Acrid Discharges.

16. Pains in places where the bones are least covered, as tibia, backs of hands, etc. (Rhus ven.).

17. Right Sided Frozen Shoulder.

18. Migraine in women who menstruate freely; excessive pains with bilious vomiting.

19. Headache begins in occiput, spreads upwards and settles over right eye; > by perfect quiet and sleep.

20. SUDDEN STOPPING OF CATARRH OF RESPIRATORY TRACT FOLLOWED BY DIARRHEA.

21. Before menses, itching of axillae.

22. WORSE by sweets, right side, motion, touch.

23. Lying on right side was impossible.

24. Rising from lying causes vertigo.

25. Cancer, Polyps, and New growths.

26. Sitting up and passing flatus ameliorates cough.

27. MENSES: AMENORRHOEA: PULMONARY DISEASE, WITH.

28. Severe burning in stomach; vomits bitter water and sour acrid fluids; nausea not relieved by vomiting.

29. Sweets aggravate the burning; vomiting of worms; tormenting thirst; sweets taste bitter.

30. Aversion to butter; craving piquant things; Unquenchable thirst.

31. Painful enlargement of breasts.

32. Sensation as if hot water were poured from breast into abdomen.
33. Pain in right breast extends to shoulder, can hardly place hand on head.
34. Cancer of the breast with severe burning pains; inflammatory symptoms of the mucous membranes of the respiratory and gastrointestinal tracts and the skin.
35. MAMMAE: SENSITIVE: TOUCH, SORE TO, UNDER RIGHT NIPPLE.
36. Mammae: stitches.
37. MAMMAE: STITCHES: PIERCING PAIN, SHARP, IN RIGHT, BENEATH NIPPLE.
38. Nipples: Burning, Sore.

21. Sarsaparilla Officinalis

Sarsaparilla is a weed from Liliaceae Family.

It is a damage tolerant plant capable of growing back from its rhizomes after being cut, burnt or frozen.

It contains Steroids which exhibit action like Glucocorticoids, Testosterone and Progesterone.

Due to presence of these Phytosteroids, it is used to build up the body and also as a natural supplement of testosterone and progesterone.

It's a well proven remedy in a recent research for cytotoxic and anti-apoptotic properties and for treatment of cancer.[26]

Glucocorticoids and Testosterone are capable to damage and destroy kidneys , presented by ample of symptoms of renal pathology in this remedy.

The presence of Progesterone makes it a remedy for Endometriosis and **Progesterone Positive Breast Cancer,** Progesterone influences breasts and causes dimpling, peu de' orange appearance of skin with Inversion/Retroversion of Nipples, producing pathology similar to **Paget's Disease.**

Combined action of Corticoids and Progesterone makes it indicated for **Inflammatory kind of Breast Cancer** as well.

Presence of excessive progesterone reduces estrogen, as a result, skin becomes rough, dry and prone to various eruptions, especially before menses.

Progesterone also produces sadness and gloominess affecting neurochemicals which is also a characteristic symptom of Sarsaparilla, having pain accompanied by gried every time and not seen in any other remedy.

Keywords: Progesterone; Testosterone; Glucocorticoids; Nephrotoxic; Peu D' Orange, Paget's Disease; Skin Symptoms related to Menses; PR + Breast Cancer

Homeopathic Indications

1. For dark - haired persons, Lithic or Sycotic diathesis.
2. Great emaciation; skin becomes shriveled or lies in folds.
3. Anxiety accompanies the pains of Sars., and the pains causes depression.
4. Herpetic eruptions.
5. Rhagades: skin cracked burning, hard, indurated.
6. Fig warts.
7. Neither appetite nor thirst, the thought of food is disgusting.
8. Ulcers, cutaneous eruptions, nodes, indurated glands, caries, necrosis, articular swellings, and rheumatism.
9. WORSE, dampness at night, after urinating, when yawning, in spring, before menses.
10. Stone formation in kidneys and bladder with painful. dysfunction of those organs; can pass urine freely only in a standing position.

11. SEVERE PAIN AT CONCLUSION OF URINATION. URINE DRIBBLES WHILE SITTING.
12. MENSES: RETARDED: URGING TO URINATE, PRECEDED BY.
13. Itching eruption on forehead during menses (Eug. j., Sang., Psor.).
14. Moist eruption in right groin before menses.
15. Menses late, scanty, acrid excoriating inside of thighs, preceded by frequent desire to urinate.
16. Climacteric Period.
17. Abortion: disposition to.
18. Intolerable stench on genital organs.
19. Retractions of nipples; nipples are small, withered, unexcitable (Sil.).
20. Retraction of the nipples is a suspicious sign even when there is no appearance of tumor, and Sars. is helpful in patients of cancerous history when this condition is present.
21. Scirrhous Cancer of the breast.
22. Suppuration of breasts.
23. Mammae: atrophy.
24. NIPPLES: WILTED. (0>1>0)

22. Scrophularia Nodosa

C.N.: Knotted Figwort. Scrophula denotes Throat. The flowers of plant resemble throat, so it is believed to treat throat ailments and has remained a medicine of repute to treat various conditions with enlarged lymph nodes of neck region as well as various types of Cancers amongst herbalists.

It is a kind of parasitic plant, which survives on the process called "HAUSTORIA". In botany and mycology, a **Haustorium** is a root-like structure that grows into or around another structure to absorb water or nutrients. In botany, this may refer to the root of a parasitic plant (such as the broomrape family or mistletoe) that penetrates the host's tissue and draws nutrients from it. In mycology, it refers to the appendage or portion of a parasitic fungus, which performs a similar function.

Another, such famous parasitic plant is Mistletoe. Both Scrophularia and Mistletoe are interestingly known for their anti-cancer properties.

In nature also, a pathogen which behaves exactly in similar fashion is "FUNGI".

The homeopathic symptomatology of this remedy is rich with various kind of skin eruptions such as Ringworm which can be attributed to fungus infection to various autoimmune diseases like Pemphigus, SLE and Lymphoma.

Recent studies in mycology has confirmed the role of mycotoxins produced by Aspergilli and Fusarium species (they also survive through the process of '**Haustoria**') responsible for cancer. **Aflatoxin** is responsible for various lung, liver and Gatrointestinal cancers while **Zearalenone** from Fusarium Fungus produces Estrogen derivatives and is linked with Hormone positive Breast Cancer, especially in African regions where the grains and water sources are highly contaminated with Molds.[27]

Aspergilli and Fusarium are also top-ranking fatal infections in neutropenic stage of lymphoma, especially of T cell origin.

Scrophularia extracts are found to relive proliferation and infiltration of T cell lymphoma.

From these scientific data and homeopathic provings, it can be concluded that Scrophularia Nodosa is a remedy for Estrogen Positive Breast Cancer with a strong history of fungal diseases, autoimmune disorders and T-Cell Lymphoma.[28]

Keywords: Haustoria; Fungus; Zearalenone; T Cell Lymphoma; Estrogen Positive Breast Cancer

Homeopathic Indications

1. It contains much oxalate and carbonate of lime, as well as Magnesia and Silica.
2. Despondency, much troubled about the past, and very apprehensive about the future.
3. Delusion object appear on closing eyes.
4. Troubles as after much weeping.
5. Cutting pains in articulations, like in Rhus tox, but more intense and longer-lasting, worse by rest and in open air, better in warm room, darting from knee to ankle-joints, which feel stiff.
6. Extreme drowsiness.
7. Loss of appetite with nausea.
8. History of Ringworm or other Skin Eruptions.
9. Itching of Hands.
10. Family History of Tuberculosis.
11. Asthmatic Problem; has to sit up.
12. < from lying on right side.
13. Pain in whole right lung on deep inspiration leading to cough without expectoration.
14. Cannot stand; weakness like Stannum Metallicum.
15. Enlarged Glands and Scrofulous Swelling (Cistus Can.).
16. Hard swelling like in Cistus.
17. Recurring Mastitis with Painful Hemorrhoids.
18. Nodosities in the breast.
19. Hodgkin's Lymphoma.
20. Breast tumor with metastasis to lung and liver.
21. Specific affinity for the breast, dissipating tumors after Con. fails.

23. Sempervivum Tectorum

It is from the same family of Sedum Acre and Repens, **stone crop**, grows on really **shallow surface** like rocks, etc.

It has got succulent leaves, can survive hard, extreme weather and trampling. Its name itself suggest **'live forever'**. **The Doctrine of Signature coincides exactly with latest scientific research as Sempervivum is found to induce apoptosis and autophagy in cancer cells trending towards immortality.**

It has **Piperidine** alkaloid which makes it to be used as a substitute of pepper. It also possess anti-inflammatory properties. This drug is found to bind to CANNABINOID RECEPTORS and alter their expressions.[29]

These receptors are found abundantly in CNS and GIT as well as are associated with immunity and hemopoiesis. These receptors are also associated with experience of bliss, appetite centers and pleasure related sensations.

Overstimulation of these centers due to overindulgence in sensory pleasures give rise to overeating-addictive tendencies, obesity, diabetes, various inflammatory conditions like irritable bowel diseases and pathologies like cancers with hypersensitive nerve endings.

They are found strongly associated with Her-2 positive Breast Cancer, Triple negative Breast Cancer and Inflammatory lesions.

In Islamic traditional medicine, Houseleek water has been recommended for dressing for malignant ulcers and the folklore also advocates the same.

It can also be applied for the **shallow ulcers** spreading on the local area, not showing any sign of healing as it happens in **Paget's disease**. It can also be used to soothe the cancer pain.

In Homeopathy, it is indicated for non-healing ulcers of mouth and hemorrhoids.

Keywords: Piperidine alkaloids; Cannabinoid Receptors; Her 2/ Triple Negative Breast Cancer; Paget's Disease, Shallow ulcers, Hemorrhoids

Homeopathic Indications

1. Ulcerated, malignant cancer, bleeding easily specially at night.
2. Flushed surface, stinging pain.
3. Too exalted vascular activity.
4. Climaxes.
5. Menses, suppressed.
6. Tongue, indurations of.
7. Aphthae, Herpes zoster, warts and corns, ringworm.

24. Solanum Mamosum

It's a plant from Solanaceae (tomato, potato, tobacco) family, also known as Nipple fruit, Sodom's apple, etc because of the shape of fruits resembling human nipple and cow's udder.

This plant is an agricultural weed.

The juice of this plant is natural detergent.

The fruits have hallucinogenic and toxic properties.

In ancient times, the juice of this plant was used to treat cracked nipples and breast abscess.

It is a source of Solasodine, a poisonous, teratogenic, alkaloidal steroid compound, which is a precursor to pharmaceutical production of contraceptive pills.

Chronic administration of Solasodine produces testicular lesions resulting in a severe impairment of spermatogenic elements.

Solasodine administration in dogs also rendered the male infertile, as evident by the absence of sperms in the cauda epididymis.

This proves that this medicine has an anti-androgenic/testosterone property which will lead to excessive estrogen production. Recent studies have reported that Solasodine has powerful anticancer properties and is found to reduce the growth of Breast Cancer cell lines.[30]

The ability of this drug to reduce androgen makes it suitable for patients having history of oophorectomy, oral contraceptive intake, adrenal gland and pituitary tumors, and menopause.

Patients present with the symptoms of obesity, low sex drive, reduced muscle tone, fatigue, large breasts and decreased bone mass due to decreased testosterone level.

Keywords: Solasodine, Anti Androgen, Excessive Estrogen, Hormone Positive Breast Cancer

Homeopathic Indications

1. Similar to Belladonna.
2. Sensitiveness to tobacco (Ign.).
3. Dreams of death with violent weeping.
4. < by flood tide, full moon.
5. > Ebb Tide (marked moon phases).
6. Hawking of blood.
7. Metastasis to lungs.
8. Left hip joint Pain< walking; > standing, sitting.
9. Swelling of mammary gland with profuse secretion of milk.
10. Profuse white leucorrhea.
11. Becomes exasperated at things he think to happen.
12. Desire to sleep with inability to sleep.
13. Difficulty in thinking and expressing ideas.

25. Taxus Baccata

Family: Coniferae (Thuja family).

C.N.: Yew.

This is one of the most ancient, long-lived but highly toxic trees. Every part including seeds and cut foliage except the red, sweet aril around the seeds are extremely toxic.

This plant possesses an extraordinary ability to survive extreme situations and plant pathogens giving it longevity. Till date, 5000 years old trees are still alive and are recorded.

These defense, fitness and survival of such plant species are attributed to their mutual relationships with plant endophytes.

Endophytes are varied species of microbes which share mutualism with plants, which provide them carbon and other nutrients, and in return, endophytes like fungi and bacteria produce biochemical metabolites which protect plants from pathogens and herbivores, making them resistant to unfavorable circumstances and adaptable to survive the extreme circumstances.

These endophytic metabolites are responsible for the toxicity of plants. Endophytes not only produce cytotoxins by themselves but also induce vertical changes in plant genomes that plant cells happen to alter their own biochemistry. They start producing toxins by themselves including their seeds, which are also rendered toxic.

These endophytes borne toxins are steroids, terpenes, saponins, taxanes and can be cytotoxic, antibacterial, antifungal, anti-diabetic and Teratogenic in nature. They are, most of the times, are responsible for medicinal properties and active alkaloids of plants.

Few Antibiotics like Penicillin, Cephalosporins and Chemotherapeutic drugs like Paclitaxel, Podophyllaxin and Vincristine are examples of such endophytic metabolites.

Paclitaxel and Docetaxel are one of the most potent Chemotherapeutic drugs derived from bark, needles and foliage of plant, Taxus Baccata, as well as from the culture of endophytic fungus of same species.

These drugs bind with microtubules of cell giving them stability and polymerization and thus prevents further mitosis which leads a cell ultimately to Apoptosis.

They are indicated as non-adjuvant and adjuvant chemotherapy for **Herceptin Positive** and other aggressive types of Breast cancers which are **highly metastatic and recurrent** in nature as curative, preventive and palliative therapy specially when the **Visceral Crisis Is Involved**.

The same can be applied to their Homeopathic indications to combat the side effects of crude drug in chemotherapeutically treated patients.

Taxus Baccata is not a well-proven drug but its side effects; are well documented; are listed which will be the authentic indications for its prescription.

Amongst them, one of the noteworthy side effects is fluid retention. Conifers are water loving plants, can store water to survive the extreme. Thuja of same family is also well known for its Hydrogenic nature. These together implies Visceral or Generalized Edema as one of the leading indications of T. Baccata.

Poisoning of T. Baccata includes hypotension and fatal cardiac dilation due to action of its cardiac glycosides over sodium pump and calcium ion channel, quite similar to Sanguinaria, and also produces action similar to Acute Adrenalin crisis. The chronic effects can be seen due to prolonged stress resulting into hypertension, palpitation and altered levels of Reactive Oxygen Stress at molecular levels giving rise to various malignancies.

Side effects of chemotherapeutic drugs extracted from this plant show the following characteristic indications:

1. Low blood counts.
2. Hair loss.
3. Arthralgias and myalgias,
4. Peripheral neuropathy.
5. Nausea and vomiting.
6. Diarrhea.
7. Mouth sores.
8. Hypersensitivity reaction. Fever, facial flushing, chills, shortness of breath, or hives.
9. Swelling of the feet or ankles (edema).
10. Increases in blood tests measuring liver function.
11. Low blood pressure.
12. Darkening of the skin.
13. Nail changes (discoloration of nail, brittleness).

Homeopathic Indications

1. Rumbling, Gurgling with empty stomach.
2. Extreme hopelessness.
3. Intolerance of Hunger < Morning.
4. Thuja-like symptoms.
5. Empty feeling in stomach; must eat frequently.
6. Cough causes headache.
7. Cough < Deep Inspiration.
8. < before and after each meal; after coition.
9. Right Sided headache with lachrymation.

26. Thuja Occidentalis

Thuja is from the same family, Coniferae, and is indicated for breast cancer. Its action is similar to that of Taxus.

Homeopathic Indications

1. Left Sided.
2. Oily Face.
3. Chilliness.
4. Cauliflower-like growth.
5. History of Immunization.
6. Urging or stools after breakfast or tea.
7. Onions disagree.
8. Burning.
9. Varicose veins during menstruation.
10. Localized perspiration.
11. Perspiration on uncovered parts.
12. Brown spots on skin.
13. Difficulty in eating vegetables and fruits.
14. Allergy.
15. Desires salt.
16. < Sun.
17. Dreams falling from a height.
18. Teeth are serrated, yellow in color.
19. Faulty.
20. Persistent Insomnia.
21. Frequent urination with pain.
22. Sweats copiously on going to sleep, one constantly moves and turns in bed, and is worse keeping still.
23. Tumors, growths, warts, moles.
24. H/o recurrent UTI.

27. Trifolium Pratensis

Family: Leguminosae (Pea/Baptisia Family); C.N.: Red Clover.

Parts used: Flowering buds.

This plant is used in many medicinal schools since beginning for the treatment of whooping cough, hay's asthma and bronchitis.

The flower buds are used as an external application for cancerous growth.

In many experiments, it has been found useful to control breast cancer and induce apoptosis.

It contains flavonoid, Coumarin, which is a Phytoestrogen and a potential medicine for Estrogen Positive Breast Cancer. It is found to affect Beta Estrogen Receptors which produce malignancy, inducing apoptosis of breast cancer cells.

After studying hundreds of research papers, it can be deduced that the Coumarin present in the Trifolium acts as an anticoagulant like Warfarin. It acts on the Vascular Endothelial Growth Factors (VGEF), their Receptors and Angiogenesis needed for the tumor formation.

Thus, increased presence of VGEF markers in blood sera is a reliable indication to prescribe Trifolium Pretense for Estrogen Positive Breast Cancer.

As a member of legume family, it also presents a feeling of confusion/being scattered in thoughts and/or action at mental level.

Keywords: Coumarin; Phytoestrogen; VGEF; Estrogen Positive Breast Cancer

Homeopathic Indications

1. PRODUCES MOST MARKED PTYALISM.

2. Feeling as if mumps were coming on.
3. Confusion and headaches on awaking. Dullness in anterior brain. Mental failure, loss of memory.
4. Sore throat, with hoarseness.
5. HOARSE AND CHOKING; CHILLS WITH COUGH AT NIGHT. Cough on coming into the open air.
6. Neck stiff; cramp in sterno-cleido muscles; relieved by heat and irritation.
7. Cough followed by hiccough.
8. Sensation in lungs as if breathing hot air, as if air full of impurities.
9. "Sharp pain through uvula causing tears to start." Dryness of trachea causing him to clear throat of some foreign substance.
10. Painless menstruation.
11. Cancerous Diathesis.
12. Retards progress of cancerous tumors before ulceration has taken place.

Chapter 5

Animal Remedies

1. Apis Mellifica

Common Name: Western Honeybee.

Honeybee is an industrious insect, woven with human life since centuries.

Honeybee lives in a well-organized complex female dominating society based on caste, sex, genetic predominance and work distribution according to aging. This organization is headed by a Queen Bee and comprises worker bees and drones.

Drones can be laid by bee without fertilization, while to lay female eggs, a bee require fertilization.

In a colony of thousands of bees, only one Queen exists who plays a central role in maintenance and survival of entire colony. Only Queen Bee has right to mate with drones and lay fertilized eggs for colony. She is Polyandrous (mating more than one male, sometimes the number crosses 50) by nature, intensely mates with drones during the season, stores spermatozoa in her special sacs and lays eggs over the time. As worker bees have no sexual right, they are engaged in the activities of building, cleaning nests; nursing and rearing eggs; finding and storing food, and defense.

Few larvae are fed with Royal jelly to develop into a queen bee.

A stronger young queen bee kills all her sisters after her elder mother queen leaves the hive, kills the drones after mating and her eggs are policed by worker bees to eggs laid by other worker bees; there is a tremendous hierarchy. She is rightly called one of the most jealous organisms.

A Queen's power is defined by her ability to get fertilized and secrete pheromones, i.e. it lies in her endo- and exocrine glands. There are mystic chemicals secreted by bees which governs major aspects of their life cycle.

Pheromones secreted by queen are very much desired by worker bees. They go in her proximity to rub their bodies, lick her and are very much essential to the extent that they cannot exist without. A queen with more potent ovaries and more fertilized eggs is found more attractive. But these varied pheromones suppress the development of ovaries in worker bees due to which they can never get fertile. A difference in Queen and worker Bee is mere development of ovaries.

During the homoeopathic drug proving, the medicinal action is also found centered around skin, genitourinary tract and ovaries. It is a good remedy for PCOD, Infertility and Ovarian and Breast Cancer. This shows that it might have more likelihood to treat **Breast and Ovary Cancer Syndrome** which include hormone positive breast cancers, seen in families with BRCA 1 and 2 gene mutations present. BRCA gene is necessary for repair of damaged DNA strands and its mutation is found associated with cancers associated with Ovary and Breast; is hereditary in nature.

Melittin, a main peptide of Bee Venom, is proven as a promising painkilling and anticancer agent in various experiments.[31] The highly inflammatory nature of bee venom exhibited during drug proving makes Apis Mellifica a potent medicine for Inflammatory Breast Cancer as well.

Keywords: Female Domination, Hierarchy, Jealousy, Ovaries, Hormone Positive, BRCA Mutations, Inflammatory

Homeopathic Indications

1. Stinging, burning pain; suddenly migrating from one part to another.
2. Hypersensitivity.
3. Scirrhus growth, open ulcers.
4. Prolonged and Obstinate Constipation.
5. Threatened Abortion Specially During first trimester of pregnancy.
6. Thirstless.
7. Hot.
8. Tendency for visceral dropsies with swelling under lower eye lids; pale, waxy, almost transparent.
9. DEATH: ANTICIPATION OF: SUDDEN, IN PERITONITIS.
10. Women, especially widows; children and girls who, though generally careful, become awkward, and let things fall while handling them (Bov.).
11. Ailments from jealousy, fright, rage, vexation, bad news.
12. Irritable; nervous; fidgety; hard to please.
13. Weeping disposition; cannot help crying; discouraged, despondent (Puls.).
14. Sexual excitement: Nymphomania.
15. PREGNANCY: ABDOMEN: TIGHT, SENSATION AS IF SOMETHING, WOULD BREAK IF TOO MUCH EXERTION WERE MADE AT STOOL.
16. MENSES: SHORT DURATION, OF: OVARIAN TUMOR, LAST A DAY OR TWO, IN.
17. OVARIES: HEAVINESS: MAMMAE, IN OVARIAN DROPSY AND CANCER OF.
18. OVARIES: TUMORS: CYST, SIZE OF A HEAD.
19. Nipples: retracted: inverted.
20. MAMMAE: CANCER: BURNING: OF OPEN.

2. Asterias Rubens

It is a well-known homeopathic remedy for Breast Cancer, derived from starfish.

During a research, it was found that polysaccharides of starfish could cure cancer cells by inhibiting the COX 2 pathway and reducing the Prostaglandin synthesis.[32]

Overexpression of COX 2 pathway and excessive prostaglandin synthesis is one of the responsible factors for Breast malignancy. Chronic Injuries/Inflammation, Stressors, Hormonal imbalances and few unknown factors lead to overexpression of COX 2 pathway.

This pathway is rightly called "Phoenix Rising Pathway" in which injuries to cancer cells due to surgery and radiation lead to revived aggressive expression signals, resulting in regrowth of malignant tumors, thus proving cancer to be unbeatable in spite of ultra-scientific surgeries, chemotherapy and radiations.[33]

Inhibiting the COX 2 pathway without side effects is a big challenge.

But the starfish seems to hold the promise of this therapeutic efficacy.

The COX 2 pathway is active during embryonic state, works over stem cells and is responsible for the abundant growth potential and fetal respiration in amniotic fluid. It is also associated with induction of labor, helping out in prostaglandin production required for cervical dilatation and other events. It gets deactivated after birth.

Malignant tumor behaves like an embryo and Cancer cells behave like stem cells. COX 2 is responsible for the abundant growth, inflammatory reactions and invasion of Cancerous tissues.

Starfish is very primitive organism made up of undifferentiated stem cells of Pluripotent type (attributing to capacity to regrow an amputed limb or becoming individual organisms from two cut halves) surviving million years of challenges under the sea, like an Embryo. Single starfish can lay 2.5 million egg at a time. Research has confirmed that a pathway similar to COX and prostaglandins are responsible for Enormous Fecundity, Ability to Breath under the Sea and Autonomy in Asterias.

A research study has also proved that chemo-preventive efficacy of polysaccharides obtained from starfish in progression and metastasis of cancer and starfish extract is found to be more effective than current Tamoxifen in treating Hormone positive Breast Cancer.

Keywords: COX 2 and Prostaglandin; Phoenix Rising Pathway; Stem Cells: Embryo-Starfish-Cancer Tumor; Starfish Polysaccharides; Estrogen Positive Breast Cancer

Homeopathic Indications

1. For the Sycotic diathesis; flabby, lymphatic constitution; irritable temperament.

2. Easily excited by any emotion, especially contradiction; epilepsy.

3. Weeps from least emotion which relieves.

4. Hallucinations; of hearing voices; away from; among strangers. (Schizophrenia).

5. Sense of impending misfortune. Afraid of bad news.

6. Sensation as if the whole head is surrounded by an atmosphere of hot air.

7. Intense throbbing of carotid arteries.

8. A picture of apoplexy, epilepsy, hysteria, chorea, neuralgia.

9. Increase of the venereal appetite about the early hours of the morning making the patient ill - humor and hysterical throughout the day.

10. IDEAS: CLEAR, AFTER HEADACHE.

11. IDEAS: VIOLENCE, OF, PRODUCED BY IMPORTUNATE VENEREAL CRAVING.

12. Unusual moisture of the vagina, which affords relief.

13. Severe general pain over the womb, as if something protruded behind it.

14. Loss of appetite. Uncertain appetite. Dullness of taste.

15. Aversion to meat.

16. Desires cold drinks, highly seasoned food, strong cheese, liquors, tea.

17. Constipation: obstinate; ineffectual desire; stools of hard, round balls, like olive.

18. Worse: Heat. Menses. Contradiction. Cold wet weather. Coffee. Night.

19. Numerous cases are on record where Asterias brought not only palliation but a radical cure of cancer of mammae even in the ulcerative stage.

20. Cancer of the left breast.

21. Miliary or ferulaceous eruption between the breasts.

22. Blotch on the chest as large as a child's palm, causing a great deal of itching.

23. Drawing pain towards the inner portion of the chest from before backward; under the left breast, which extends over the whole inner portion of the arm to the end of the little finger.

24. Cancer of mammae; around nipple, which is sunk in, skin adherent and smooth; livid red spot which ulcerates, discharging very fetid ichor; pale, hard, everted edges; swollen and painful sternal skin; axillary glands swollen, hard and knotted.

3. Badiaga

Common name: Freshwater Sponge; Spongilla lacustris

Sponge is made up of Silica, Lime and Alumina and is rich source of Iodine. They play a vital role in ecology by filtering water reservoirs inhabited by them.

Fresh water sponges face tougher condition to survive than marine ones which led to development of "**Gemmules**" to **survive by means of dormancy,** the result of asexual reproduction.

They can lie dormant for pretty long time and are resistant to **desiccation, freezing and anoxia,** then they grow into new sponge when condition becomes less hostile.

Sponges are one of the most ancient primitive organisms dating before Jurassic Time, estimated around older than 800 million years.

They have adapted to the most challenging situations, survived the toughest and developed strong biological defense against various kinds of predators. They also have a capacity to regenerate themselves.

Scientists have discovered the most promising kind of antiviral/ bacterial/fungal as well anticancer molecules from sponges.

In fact, sponges are discovered to have those ancient genes which helps them to survive but are responsible for carcinogenesis in humans. Similar to Asterias, these primitive marine creatures are also stem cells and a malignant tumor too is made up of cancer stem cells, thus both share similar genetic expressions and pathways for their growth/proliferation.

FER, a protein kinase gene, is responsible for cell adhesion and signaling, is found useful for defense and survival in sponges, and the same **FER** molecular pathway is found helpful in few cancers including breast, as blocking them resulted into tumor suppression.[34]

This **FER T pathway** is found associated with basal/triple negative and highly metastatic kind of Breast Cancer and Badiaga is also one of the medicines to correct this pathway, thus a medicine for the above mentioned breast malignancy.

Badiaga is an excellent cosmetic medicine for Acne Rosacea/ vulgaris, photo-dermatitis and many skin pathologies like psoriasis .

Keywords: Silica+Alumina+ Calcium+ Iodine; FER T Pathway; Basal like Breast Cancer; Skin Pathologies

Homeopathic Indications

1. General soreness of the muscles and skin as if beaten.

2. Hyperesthesia of muscles and integuments; worse motion and friction of clothes.

3. Mucus flies out from mouth and nostrils.

4. < by cold, stormy weather, pressure; > by heat.

5. Metrorrhagia < at night with feeling of enlargement of head.

6. Injuries: Concussion: Lesions, Pains and Suggillations.

7. Swelling: Hard, Convolute, Glandular.

8. Emotion: palpitation, causes pleasurable, from. (3>2>0)

9. Mental Activity: Headache, In Spite of.

10. Weeping: cough: during.

11. Strumous and hemorrhoidal persons with pulmonic and cardiac symptoms.

12. Skin: Freckles and Rhagades.

13. Cancer: Mammae (pulmonic constitution suggests tendency to metastasis to lungs).

4. Bufo Rana

This medicine is prepared from the poisonous secretion from the skin and parotid like gland of Common Toad. Toads were introduced in many regions to control the pest but now have become an **invasive, prolific** species and act as a **pest**.

The poison is secreted by the parotid glands when the frog is threatened, and is used as an **"Aphrodisiac"**, **Psychedelic** drug. It can prove to be fatal, therefore was also used as an **arrow poison**.

Schizophrenics, autistic, OCD and paranoid offenders' urine samples are found to contain more **Bufotenine** than normal.

This secretion produces drooling of saliva, brick-red mucous membrane, epilepsy and death due to cardiac failure in the victim with presence of steroidal cardiac glucosides and other bufotoxins.

This lipid soluble secretion, injected into cancer patients, is an official medicine "Huachansu" of Cancer in Chinese medicine and is validated useful in various clinical trials of multidrug resistant cancer affecting multiple cancer-causing molecular pathways (for Liver, Lungs, Blood, Breast, etc.) . The cardiac toxin works like Digitalis and deters Na^+P^+ Pump while other toxins are anti-inflammatory and highly anti-cancerous.

Toad performs external conception during the process of copulation, a male toad mounts the back of a female and rubs his genitalia on her back holding her with front legs, sometimes for couple of days, and female lays 8000-25,000 eggs at a time. An over-enthusiastic frog mounts back of a fish, wood or male frog sometimes to release himself of his sexual needs and this natural behavior explains the reason why Bufo Rana is one of the top-ranking medicines for tendency to masturbate in Homeopathy and used as an aphrodisiac drug.

Most of the times, male toads outnumber females and many toads mounts her back at a time. The female frog is literally gang raped, mounted over by number of toads even after getting crushed and dead for long period finally consumed by the spawned and fertilized eggs of her own.

This aspect portrays the syphilitic aspect of this remedy and points towards Cancer of Breast in females with chronic history of sexual/ mental/ emotional abuse or assault; inflammatory; hormone positive as well as metastatic and aggressive in nature.

This behavior and hallucinogenic properties also indicate a kind of sexual-minded offender, grown physically but underdeveloped intellectually and morally, who cannot hold his sexuality and could be a patient of a serious mental disease like Paranoia, Schizophrenia, OCD, Autism or other growth disorders.

This venom produces epilepsy, and is useful for epilepsy related to sexuality and menstruation.

The brick red discoloration of affected part by this venom is also a strong indication when chosen for malignant inflammation.

Keywords: Huachansu[35], Brick Red Mucous Membrane; Drooling, OCD, Autism, Addiction, Schizophrenia, Paranoia; Rape, Cardiac Effects, Epilepsy, Inflammatory and Hormone Positive Breast Cancer[36]

Homeopathic Indications

1. Mentally Dwarf, Sexually Developed.
2. Addiction tendencies
3. Arouses the lowest passions.
4. Desire for Solitude. Feeble-Minded.
5. Overindulgence in sex with epilepsy.
6. Epilepsy during sleep, menses, coition.
7. Great weakness of memory; idiotic; extremely sensitive to light and noise.
8. Music unbearable.

9.   Anger: Understood, When Incoherent Speech Is Not.

10. Lymphangitis of septic origin.

11. Induration of Mammary Gland; open and occult cancer.

12. Mastitis, purulent sinuses; sensation as if breasts were torn towards abdomen.

13. Bloody milk/lactation.

14. Palliative in breast cancer.

15. Late cancer, removes fetor in helpless case of cancer.

16. Terminal Stage of Cancer.

17. Induration of Mammary Gland.

5. Castoreum Equi

Castoreum Equi is prepared from Rudimentary Thumb-nail of the Horse. It has been prove useful for swollen, sensitive breasts with excessive tenderness.

Homeopathic Indications

1.   "The rudimentary thumb-nail of the horse".

2.   This is an ancient remedy and was proved and introduced into homeopathy by Hering. It especially acts on nipples, nails, bones, especially causing pains in right tibia and coccyx; Nails drop off.

3.   General action on thickening of the skin and epithelium.

4.   Dental Caries; PAIN: IN LEFT SIDE: CARIOUS, MUST PICK THEM.

5.   Hysteria; Unusual laughter about things not funny.

6.   Facial Warts.

7.   Warts on breast. Chapped hands.

8.   Breasts swollen, sensitive, itching internally, painful on descending stairs.

9. Nipples Ulcerated, in nursing mothers; cannot bear touch of clothing.

10. MAMMAE: HEAVINESS: FEEL AS THOUGH THEY WOULD FALL OFF, SHE MUST PRESS HANDS AGAINST THEM.

11. MAMMAE: SWELLING: PAINFUL ON DESCENDING STAIRS.

12. MAMMAE: SWELLING: RIGHT, ESPECIALLY, PAINFUL TO TOUCH.

13. MAMMAE: ITCHING: INTERNAL, DRIVING TO DESPAIR, RUBBING AND SCRATCHING BETTER, BUT MAKES SKIN ROUGH.

14. NIPPLES: AREOLA: RED, AS IN ERYSIPELAS.

15. NIPPLES: SENSITIVE: TENDER, EXCESSIVELY, CANNOT.

16. NIPPLES: ULCERS: NEARLY ULCERATED OFF, HANGING BY STRINGS.

17. Paget's Disease.

6. Lac Canninum

Nothing noteworthy is known about the medicinal properties of Bitch's milk and its role in treatment of cancer, but Lac Canninum is listed as a remedy for Breast Cancer, especially when it develops in left mammae after the surgical removal of same from the right breast.

A bitch is a mammal and undergoes estrous cycle, lactate like humans and also prone to mastitis and Breast Cancer. Milk production in Bitch is also associated with a complex hormonal cycle and psychological state of her.

The homeopathic proving denotes it as a head remedy for assisting weaning, galactorrhea, agalactia and Diabetes mellitus, acting over Pituitary by axis of Growth Hormone-Prolactin-Insulin like

Growth Factors which control growth of breast, lactogenesis and cessation of lactation. The same axis when altered produces Galactorrhea, large breast size, Atrophy of Breast in secondary action, Diabetes Mellitus and Breast Cancer with IGF 2 Receptors overexpressed. (DDx Chimaphilla Umbellata)

Generally, this remedy acts more over Herceptin Positive Breast Cancer.

In Homeopathy, Lac Canninum is indicated for its action over chronic tonsillitis and mastitis as both the infections are associated with

Staphylococcus Aureus, which can also be one of the clinical confirmations to prescribe Lac Canninum for Breast Cancer.

Keywords: Pituitary; Growth Hormone; Prolactin; Diabetes Mellitus; Galactorrhea; IGF 2; HER 2 Positive Breast Cancer

Homeopathic Indications

1. Alternating Sides.
2. Complementary to Lachesis.
3. Delusion and Fear of snakes; rope on the floor which seems like a snake.
4. Intolerance of picture of Snake even in TV or Photo.
5. Extreme Forgetfulness.
6. Loathing of Life.
7. Miserable; Feels "I am not worthy of medicine".
8. Chronic Blue Condition.
9. Erratic pain shifting from side to side.
10. Very Hungry, as hungry as before eating.
11. Very prominent throat symptom.
12. An antidote to deadly poisons.
13. Corners of mouth and alae nasi cracked.

14. Pains come and leave quickly.

15. Migraine.

16. Nutrition: Defective, Causes Swollen, Ulcerated, Retracted, Bleeding Gums and Loose Teeth.

17. "Inflamed surfaces glistening".

18. Sensation of lightness or levitation, feel as if walking on air, cannot touch the bed when lying.

19. Wants to lie with her knees to her chin.

20. Cannot bear one part of her body to touch another, must even keep her fingers apart.

21. Walking causes leucorrhea, worse sores between labia and thighs.

22. Worse by Touch (external throat, breasts) causing sexual excitement.

23. Menses: bright red blood, forms into long strings when put in water.

24. ABORTION: SEQUELAE: BREASTS, KNOTS AND CAKES IN.

25. ABORTION: TIME: SIX MONTHS.

26. After the amputation of breast, other side of breast is affected.

27. First one breast is involved, then the other.

28. Breast Painful < Least Jar; Must hold like Bryonia.

29. GLANDS: SWELLING: LYMPHATIC, ALTERNATE SIDE.

30. NIPPLES: PAIN: CONSTANT.

7. Lachesis Muta

C.N. Bushmaster, Surukuku, Pit Viper.

This is one of the South American deadliest and longest vipers.

The venom is highly hemotoxic and neurotoxic by nature.

Much is known about its toxicology and homeopathic drug picture.

Most of the snake and insect venoms contain enzyme containing Phospholipase A2. The enzyme when introduced into body by snake or insect bite, produces local pain and inflammation by binding to Cytochrome C Oxidase leading to release of Arachidonic Acid, release of Prostaglandin, Interleukins and activation of COX 2 pathway.

Cytochrome C oxidase is the last enzyme of cellular respiration which functions to release energy from food particles. It is also the site for binding of various toxins, Chronic inflammatory products, molecular waste, environmental pollutants, carcinogens leading to increased Oxidative Stress which can ultimately lead to malignancy, Estrogen Positive malignancy of Breast. Hence, most of the reptiles and insect venoms are found curative in such cancers when prescribed in the basis of Law of Similars. They hold the potential to detoxify the body from chronic poisoning of above-mentioned kind and reverse the grave pathological changes.

The modern science lacks an art to administer such poisons as a curative remedy for cancer while they have already proven its potential for anticancer therapy. The other challenge is how to differentiate between clinical indications of this diverse range of cytotoxins. Homeopathic Materia Medica and its unique drug delivery system are the answer to both these challenges.

Lachesis is a secretive kind of nocturnal reptile which sits hidden merging with the environment, waiting for its prey to reach nearby, then it performs its deadliest fatal attack to capture. A pair of highly evolved thermo-sensing pits facilitates such survival strategy and makes it different from other snakes, giving it infrared vision to see at night.

According to recent findings, the thermo-sensing pits have "wasabi" or TRPA 1[37] kind of receptors attached to trigeminal ganglia which gives them nocturnal vision. These receptors are also present in humans which provides ability to feel pain sensation and heat saving from injurious stimuli. The same receptors are found overexpressed in malignancy and their blockage resulted into pain reduction and tumor regression. This data is self-explanatory that Lachesis is a cancer medicine which can treat cancer as well as inflammation and pain related to it by inhibiting overexpressed TRPA 1 Receptors.

Keywords: Secretive; Hemotoxic-Neuro Toxic; Cox 2, Detox; Estrogen Positive Breast Cancer; Nocturnal Vision; Wasabi Receptors; Cancer Pain

Homeopathic Indications

1. Left Sided Affections.
2. Symptoms go left to right.
3. Better by discharges.
4. Aggravated before Menses.
5. < Morning on waking and during sleep.
6. Intolerance of tight clothes.
7. Hot Patient.
8. Dreams or Delusion of Snakes.
9. Clairvoyance.
10. Unhappy love, with jealous, suspicious despair; weary of life; pain in heart; fainting, apparent death; mistrust, suspicion; worse towards evening.
11. Dread of death, fears to go to bed; fears she will be damned; thinks herself pursued by enemies or robbers; fears the medicine as poison; fears insanity.
12. Females approaching the fifth decade, following a period of glandular and circulatory disturbances affecting the thyroid, ovaries and liver; Vertigo, flashes of heat, palpitations, general hyperesthesia (cannot tolerate anything tied about the neck, chest or waist) and often, arterial hypertension.
13. Intoxicated (alcohol) or jaded. Its action is more general on the intoxication of cancerous origin.

14. Sensation of " a lump" or "a ball" found in the throat.

15. Chill at night and hot flushes by day.

16. Blue rings around eyes.

17. Hydrothorax, with suffocative fits, waking from sleep, with throwing the arms about; skin over the edematous parts cyanotic; black urine; offensive smell of feces; complications with heart, liver and spleen troubles.

18. Ovarian tumors, even when suppuration has taken place (after - Merc. or Hep.) when adynamia prevails.

19. Melanosis; Colloid or Encephalic Cancer, Gangrenous Spots.

20. Scattered small ulcers , with pain in old cicatrices; pain or burning in the ulcers upon being touched. The skin in the neighborhood of the tumor is of a livid or mottled appearance.

21. Breast has a bluish or purplish appearance; lancinating pains in mammae and down the arm.

22. Open cancer has a dark, bluish - red appearance, with blackish streaks of decomposed blood.

23. Coughing or sneezing causes stitches in affected parts.

24. Cancer of breast, with lancinating pains; worse in open air, from pressure, and after sleep, better in dry weather.

25. MAMMAE: FUNGUS HEMATODES: RIGHT, ON, AS LARGE AS A PEONY, BLOOD POURED OUT AS FROM A SPONGE.

26. MAMMAE: PURPLISH.

27. MAMMAE: TUMORS: THREE, LOBED, EACH LOBE AS LARGE AS A PIGEON'S EGG, TWO INCHES ABOVE AND TO LEFT OF NIPPLE, MOVABLE, AND PAINFUL TO PRESSURE, EXAMINATION CAUSES PAIN, EXTENDS TO SHOULDER AND DOWN ARM, LASTING FIVE TO SIX HOURS.

8. Murex Purpurea

Murex is made from the purple ink extract from the glands of Bolinus Bandaris, a marine snail.

The extract from the glands of snails was used by Romans and Greek to make a purple dye, 'Tyrian Purple', which was a symbol of royalty and worn only by those from very elite class.

This purple dye is squirted by a snail when attacked as a chemogenic defense, and is found in hypo-brachial gland, gonads, gut and surrounding eggs of snails as a protective layering. Snail produces and uses multiple chemicals for defense, wound healing, alarm and preying.

This purple dye is chemically a Bromo peroxidase, a rich source of indirubin, and is found to act as anti-bacterial/viral/fungal, anti-inflammatory and cytotoxic. It also acts through kinase activator, thus proving itself as a potential medicine for cancer.[40]

As the purple dye is squirted in the situation of crisis, it also contains epinephrine.

Snails are found to secrete pheromones to attract suitable sex partners and insert love hormones through a dart-like structure by piercing partner's body before and during act of copulation. They are worldwide eaten as an aphrodisiac savory. Experiments have found the extract of snails enhancing steroidogenesis and increasing sex hormones. Its homeopathic proving reflected symptoms of excessive sexual desire and nymphomania in females.

Murex is a remedy for Hormone positive Breast Cancer with excessive sexual needs, adrenalin crisis and inflammatory condition of uterus and ovaries.

Keywords: Tyrian Purple; Cytotoxic; Aphrodisiac; Adrenaline Crisis, Hormone Positive Breast Cancer

Homeopathic Indications

1. Pains are frequently diagonal and shoot from ovary to opposite breast.
2. Stitching pain in genitalia, through abdomen, up to breast.
3. Nymphomania; < by slightest touch of parts; frantic sexual desire.
4. Weakness of memory, with difficulty in finding words to express his thoughts.
5. Happier when leucorrhea is worst.
6. Leucorrhea, yellow, green or mixed with blood.
7. Better before Menses.
8. Climaxes.
9. Nightly polyuria, with the hungry craving; Diabetes.
10. Worse Night, After sleep. Must lie down from weakness but lying down worse all symptoms.
11. Distinct sensation of womb.
12. Profuse Perspiration during Menses.
13. A feeling as if something were pressing on a sore spot in the pelvis.
14. Cervix is sensitive to the examining finger.
15. The slightest touch causes bleeding of excoriation on cervix.
16. Excessive hemorrhage with large clots.
17. Violent bearing down with symptoms of prolapse, better by crossing legs.
18. Carcinoma of Uterus.
19. OVARIES: TUMORS: CYST, LARGE, SUPPOSED TO BE CONNECTED WITH LEFT OVARY, OCCUPYING SPACE BETWEEN RECTUM, UTERUS AND VAGINA, SO AS TO OBLITERATE POSTERIOR CUL DE SAC AND ALMOST OCCLUDE VAGINA.
20. Violent pains, acute lancinations in breasts.

21. Pain in chest, as if it had been bruised.
22. Lancinating and burning pains below false ribs on left side, towards back.
23. Sensation as of a snake creeping over entire region of short ribs.
24. Mammae: neuralgia.
25. Tumors of Breast.

9. Naja Tripudians

Naja, Indian Cobra, King Cobra.

This snake is worshipped in many cultures as it is linked to supernatural power and considered as a symbol of latent energy in spiritualism, possessing a mystic aura.

King Cobra is another deadliest snake which feeds mainly on other snakes. It possesses an excellent eyesight, is very agile, can attack with superfast speed and bite in rapid fire rounds. It is an aggressive and ferocious snake with very potent fatal venom but differs from other snakes by its tendency to warn before attacking and prefers to avoid confrontation at first instance.

Its venom is highly neurotoxic; cholinergic in action and cardiotoxic. It paralyzes its prey by biting before deglutition, and Homeopathic Materia Medica also describes its medicinal action centered around paralysis and heart conditions.

A Srilankan study[38] over 800 patients of snake envenomation survivors presented long-term symptoms of snake bite like migraine type of headache, tightness around chest, neuro- and myopathies, as well as hemiplegia, which are also mentioned as clinical indications in Homeopathy for this remedy.

Another study proved that this venom possess an ability to deplete Iodine from thyroid gland.[39] Iodine deficiency causes fibrocystic breast disease and is related to Estrogen positive Breast Cancer.

Cobra bite is said to produce the worst kind of pain one might not have felt ever before and is found in many studies having excellent pain-killing properties. Numerous studies have also proved its cytotoxic nature, thus helpful in controlling breast cancer lines in in-vitro studies.

Keywords: Migraine, Hemiplegia, Myo-neuropathies, Cardiac diseases; Hypothyroidism; Cancer Pain; Estrogen Positive Breast Cancer

Homeopathic Indications

1. Very Sensitive to Cold.
2. Fear of Rain.
3. Suicidal insanity.
4. Anxiety, others for.
5. Delusion, being injured by surroundings.
6. Delusion, suffered wrong.
7. Delusion, neglected duty he has.
8. Delusion, wrong, everything is.
9. Cannot endure any mental exertion.
10. Sweat over palms.
11. FOOD: Desires: Sugar, Alcohol.
12. Worse: Tobacco, Spices.
13. Better: Acid fruit, Tobacco.
14. Voracious Appetite.
15. Great dryness of the mouth. Foamed at the mouth.
16. Gloomy headache, with spinal pains and palpitations from disorders of the sexual function.
17. Sensation as if heart and ovaries were drawn together.
18. Tubercular Type.
19. Breast Lump with Cardiac Hypertrophy.
20. Intolerance of Tight Clothing.

21. Similar to Lachesis but not hemorrhagic.
22. Inability to support himself in a sitting posture.
23. For most acute pain as if a hot iron had been run in.
24. Inability to speak, with choking, nervous chronic palpitation."
25. Gasping at throat with the choking sensation.
26. TENDENCY OF ALL COMPLAINTS TO SETTLE ABOUT THE HEART.
27. Pulse slow, sometimes as slow as 45.
28. <lying on side, on left side. better of pain and breathing by lying on right side.
29. Secretion of milk very much decreased.

Note: Dr Grimmer's comment about Cancer Treatment mentioned under Naja:

"It is only in cases not too far advanced where tissue changes are not too great that a cure can be consummated with a single remedy given in a succession of potencies. Advanced cases frequently require a succession of remedies not too high in potency over much longer periods to effect cure. Cancer of the breast cured by the single remedy is not often met with; and when such results are obtained, it almost seems to belong in the realm of the miraculous."

10. Oleum Animale

C. N.: Dipple's Oil, Bone Oil.

It is a volatile coal tar-like oil obtained by **destructive distillation** of animal substances like bones, horns, etc.

Thick, viscid, brown oil having the **most repulsive odor**.

It is a **complex hydrocarbon** with nitrogen and oxygen molecule and its main constituents include Aniline, Pyrrole, Pyridine, Benzol, Picoline, etc.

Pyrrole, Pyridine, Aniline are aromatic compounds; **Pyrrole**, having nutty odor, is present in many end stage metabolites like bilirubin, biliverdin and its level is found increased in urine of Schizophrenic and Cancer patients.

It is precursor of chemotherapeutic drug, Sunitinib.

Pyridine is a precursor of many vitamins, body metabolites, having a repulsive fishy smell and anticancer medicines. It is an air-water-food pollutant, which is released by smoke of cigarettes, food, etc. and used as a solvent.

It is known to harm reproductive system in male rats.

Aniline is a dye and its derivatives are also known anticancer drugs.

These organic compounds are genotoxic, mutagenic in nature. The potent chemotherapeutic drugs made from them are anti-tubular/vasculogenic agents, which act through lysis of DNA by multiple cancer leading pathways in Leukemia, Liver, Bone and Breast Cancer.

These substances are obtained from destructive distillation of organic compounds, suggestive of an end stage pathology of tissues, breaking down into disease products and toxins with repulsive nutty, fishy, urine-like odor.

It is a medicine for recurring, metastatic, aggressive, tissue eating type of Breast Cancer involving blood, lymph, bones and other systems with foul secretion, ulceration and inflammation akin to carbons with thick, viscid, dark, acrid discharges (justifying Doctrine of Signature).

Keywords: Destruction; Repulsive Odor; Pyrrole; Pyridine; Metabolic End Toxins, Metastatic Cancer

Homeopathic Indications

1. Sad mood, morose, nothing delights her.
2. Absorbed in self, sad, speaks little.

3. "Pulled Upward and From Behind Forward" pain.

4. Stitches as with red-hot needles.

5. Left side is predominantly affected.

6. Chilly medicine, but the chilliness is worse in a warm room and better in open air.

7. Bites Cheeks while eating (Ignatia, Causticum).

8. > by Rubbing, Open Air, Pressure.

9. Profuse accumulation of snow-white saliva in mouth.

10. Eructation tastes like urine.

11. Sensation as if stomach were full of churning water.

12. Polyuria with Migraine.

13. Desire for soft-boiled eggs or for bread only with aversion to meat.

14. Yellowness of palms of hands.

15. Early and Scanty Menstruation.

16. Worse Before, during and commencement of menses.

17. Urine like leucorrhea.

18. Right Breast affected.

19. Pain, darting forward out of nipples.

11. Sepia Officinalis

Common name: Cuttlefish, Cephalopoda. Sepia is made up from the ink of cuttlefish.

This is a marine organism which has survived more than 21 million years of its existence and is the most intelligent invertebrate existing.

Sepia is also called marine chameleon as it is the king of camouflage and can change color, shape, texture, size, spots and stripes over body within seconds for the purpose of defense, mating and preying.

It has an ink sac from which it releases a reddish brown mucoid liquid mainly composed of melanin, polysaccharides, and when threatened provides a protective covering to eggs. This ink works as a blind shield between predator, sometimes forming a false image of body like a cuttlefish, to distract the predator, while most of the times, as an aversive deterrent. The ink clad fish tastes very aversive, it is a distasteful kind of food which blocks the olfactory, visual appetite centers in animals approaching them, making it a non-palatable food. It is nauseous to human taste as well.

The eggs are also covered by ink and is protects in the same way from being the tasty food of other marine organisms. This ink is also potent antimicrobial and cytotoxic in nature. It has been found as potent anti-cancer and chemo-preventive agent in many experiments.[41] It has also been found capable to reverse ovarian failure caused due to Cyclophosphamide therapy.[42]

Besides inking, Sepia camouflages to defend and attack the prey. It has ability to hypnotize other marine animals by changing shape and colors, by stunning and then paralyzes by inserting a chemical in its prey.

While mating, a male deposit its sperm in a sac near the mouth of female to fertilize but there is an extreme competition. Many times, a more powerful male captures a copulated female washing out sperms of previously mated males. A cuttlefish undergoes several cycles of such kind of induced abortion before finally hatching eggs.

The very intelligent cuttlefish in the competition to find a female plays a wonderful piece of game. Smaller sized males to overcome the larger ones camouflage themselves into sexually non receptive female cuttlefish with a typical spot over body displaying no readiness for sex and fooling the physically powerful rivals reaches the females. It is intereating that during Homeopathic Proving, Sepia is described as a Female with Male like Pelvis,

With Melanin pigments on face with no interest in sex and under Homosexuality.

The natural survival challenges and adaptation of a medicinal source can correct the similar but unnatural disease tendencies in humans.

The fish uses multiple body morphs, colors and movements to attract females. Like Tarentula, Sepia also likes Dancing and also ameliorated from it.

The prolonged survival of Sepia under depth of sea in extreme difficult conditions is due to its capacity to produce colors, polarize and reflect lights to camouflage which is governed by Melatonin Receptors in the body. Melatonin is called a Darkness hormone as it enables an organism in the absence of sunlight to defend and attack by using specialized neuromuscular sensors to produce multiple formations of color and light over the body. Sepia Ink is found to alter the melatonin secretion in experiments via complex biochemical processes.[43]

Melatonin is an important hormone produced by pineal gland in human body from evening to night after sunset. It regulates bio-rhythm; governs sleep, appetite and important hormonal cycles of body. It lowers estrogen and libido if given externally, and also induces sleep, freshness, energy, good mood and immunity against various infections. It is found as a promising agent in the treatment of breast cancer.[44]

Disruption of bio-rhythm due to sleeping late at night, staying in artificial light and in front of mobile/computer TV screen for long time especially at night, waking up late, irregular eating time, taking up hormone regulatory pills, uncontrolled sexual behavior and all modes of unnatural living habits also disrupts Melatonin production and Circadian rhythm which may lead to Malignancy.

Giving Melatonin to Breast cancer patients is found to have better treatment response.

Sepia can be a remedy for malignancy with such background and Hormone positive Breast Cancer. It seems to hold a potential to correct the overexpressed Melatonin Receptors.

Another remedy to correct hazards due to modern life is Nux Vomica which is complementary to the action of Sepia.

Keywords: Camouflage; Aversive Ink; Nausea; Melanin; Induced Abortion; Female Like Males; Dancing; Melatonin; Circadian Rhythm; Hormone Positive Breast Cancer

Homeopathic Indications

1. Pot-bellied mothers, yellow saddle across nose, irritable, faint from least exertion, leucophlegmatic constitutions.
2. Puffed, flabby persons (less frequently emaciated) with yellow or dirty yellow brown blotched skin, inclined to sweat, especially about genitals, axillae, and back, hot flushes, headache in morning, awaken stiff and tired, subject to disease of sexual organs, the general attitude is never one of strength and healthful ease, but of lax connective tissue, languor, easily produced paresis.
3. Chilly remedy due to lack of vital heat.
4. Female complaints generally, from loss of fluids, masturbation, music, milk, fat pork, during and after perspiration, during pregnancy, riding in a car, from riding on horseback, in a swing, from sexual excesses, during first hours of sleep, in snow air, from stretching the affected part, while nursing a child, from water and washing, from getting wet.
5. Coition aggravates it in both sex.
6. Ringworm on face.
7. The complexion is a dirty sallow, frequently with a yellow saddle of color across the nose.
8. Chloasma; Tell-Tale Face.
9. Weeping while telling complaints.

10. Indifference; Apathy; Great sadness and weeping, dread of being alone, of men, of meeting friends, with uterine troubles.

11. Hypochondriasis with aversion to family and to household duties.

12. Great aversion to washing.

13. Fits of uneasiness, and of hysterical spasms.

14. Sensation of a ball in inner parts, more marked in the rectum.

15. < by cold, slow motion> by vigorous exercise, dancing.

16. Weakness of the genitals; increased sex desire with frequent erections and pollutions, especially at night.

17. Homosexuality.

18. Better by Loosening clothes.

19. Lying on side, and on right side better; Lying on left side worse.

20. Losing hair after chronic headache.

21. Warts.

22. Easy benumbing of the limbs after manual labor.

23. Renewal or worse of several suffering, during and immediately after a meal.

24. Great swelling of body, with shortness of breath, without thirst.

25. Disease connected with chronic metritis.

26. Severe bearing-down pains in the uterus and rectum; Sitting with legs crossed better.

27. Tendency to abortion.

28. ABORTION: THREATENED: MONTH: FIFTH TO SEVENTH.

29. Morning sickness, vomiting of food and bile in morning, of milky fluid," "The thought of food sickens her."

30. PREGNANCY: CONSTIPATION: MANUAL ASSISTANCE MUST BE RENDERED.

31. Breast Cancer with sudden prostration, sinking, fainting
32. Swelling and suppuration of the glands.
33. Nipple crack very much across the crown in various places, ulcer very deep and sore.
34. NIPPLES: BLEEDING: SUPPURATE, SEEM ABOUT TO.
35. MAMMAE: TUMORS: SCIRRHOUS, OF RIGHT, SIZE OF HEN'S EGG, HARD, NODULATED, TENDER TO TOUCH, STINGING PAIN.

Mineral Remedies

1. Arsenic and its salts

Arsenic is a highly fatal element, tasteless, odorless and colorless in nature, mainly used by ruling class for homicidal purposes discretely. That's why, it is called 'poison of kings' and 'king of poisons.'

It produces acute as well as chronic poisoning known as Arsenicosis, due to its prolonged exposure. It disrupts ATP function by affecting citric acid cycle resulting in cell death through necrosis and increased ROS giving rise to multiple organ failure and Cancer.

It is also present in food, air, water and soil as an environmental pollutant. It is also a part of tobacco smoke. Arsenic was widely used and still used as insecticide, herbicide and pesticide. Poultry and Swine are also fed Arsenic in minor quantity for weight gain and bacterial resistance. Groundwater contamination through natural and industrial sources and presence of Arsenic in rice, apples, etc. are also major health concerns owing to its carcinogenicity.

It is a metalloid and proven class 1 Carcinogen linked with bladder, skin, kidney, blood, liver, gastric and Breast Cancer. According to the principles of Homeopathy, if a medicine can produce cancer, it can cure it as well. It is rightly listed as one of the main anticancer medicines in Homeopathic literature. Few surveys have also found that the presence of inorganic Arsenic in drinking water reduces the mortality from cancer contrary to proven scientific facts.

In fact, Arsenic Trioxide is a FDA approved medicine for acute promyelocytic leukemia (APL) and the same medicine has displayed potential role in treatment of Breast Cancer in many studies. Arsenic binds to Alpha Estrogen Receptors of Breast, thus causing and curing Breast Cancer through the same pathway. It is found to be effective against ER- negative, a highly metastatic kind of Breast Cancer also.[45]

Arsenic is being used since last 500 years as a medicine for cancer and syphilis, but the major challenge is to harness its toxicity while using in material doses. Dr Hahnemann has already solved this challenge by ultra-diluting medicinal substance and potentizing them by means of mechanical measures bringing the highest medicinal properties capable to permeate out to the deepest level, resulting in null toxic effects. Only the medical science needs a bridge to connect this wonderful discovery to the modern pharmaceutical preparations.[46]

Proving medicines on human beings is also another revolutionary discovery which enables one to differentiate one medicine from the other by finest symptomatology, and accordingly, prescribe a highly individual, genetic medicine which can bring recovery and cure to such a great level that the modern medicine still dreams about. It is a big misfortune that such discoveries have remained unacknowledged and not integrated into mainstream medicine yet.

Keywords: Arsenicosis; Carcinogen; Arsenic Trioxide; Alpha Estrogen Receptor; ER+/ER- Breast Cancer

Out of Arsenicums, Arsenic Iodatum is lesser known but has maximum affinity for Breast cancer.

Homeopathic Indications

1. Complementary to Asteria Rubens, in Carcinoma of Breast with open ulcers.
2. Extremely Hot patients with intolerance of warmth.
3. Ravenous Appetite, feels hungry even after eating.
4. Craves Meat.
5. Thin-built.
6. Hair All Over The Body.
7. Tubercular Diathesis.
8. Pale and Delicate complexion.
9. Left Sided.
10. Constant state of Hurry and Impatient.
11. Sudden impulse to kill.
12. Twitching of muscles from walking rapidly.
13. Advanced stages of diseases when Arsenic Fails.
14. Cracked and fissured tongue; offensive breath.
15. Prone to glandular affections.
16. Tendency to Diarrhea.
17. Pathology involving skin; Psoriasis, hard skin.
18. Burning sensation in nostrils, discharge thin and acrid.
19. Ulcers with thin, offensive, corrosive discharge with rapid loss of tissues.
20. Ulcerative Pain.
21. Lumps in Mammae, < by touch.
22. Nipples retracted.
23. Emaciation of Breast.
24. Violent reaction to homeopathy remedies in high potencies.

2. Aurum Metallicum and its Salts

Gold has fascinated humans since beginning of civilization for its lustrous nature and property to remain intact in its pure form. It is highly valued, and most sought among metals.

Alchemists have always believed that Gold particles give longevity because Gold doesn't rot, hence consuming it keeps the body free from decaying. This belief has led to the consumption of gold nanoparticles as medicine for various ailments and an Elixir since centuries.

Gold compounds have now emerged as promising metal based chemotherapeutic agents like Cisplatin.

They can bind to Heparin Binding Epidermal Growth Factors and alter its expression.[47] HB-EGFs are embryonic proteins associated with attachment of various phases of cell cycle, embryo attachment to endometrium, angiogenesis, neurogenesis, development of heart, wound healing, etc.

The overexpression of genes regulating these proteins is associated with Endometriosis, Atherosclerosis, Hypertrophy of Heart and other viscera, Valvular heart diseases, Rheumatoid arthritis and various kind of Malignancies. In Homeopathic proving also, similar pathological indications are presented by Aurum and its compounds.

Inhibition of HB-EGFs is proven to be effective against aggressive, metastatic hormone resistant Breast Cancer.

Thus, Aurum and its salts are useful in Breast Cancer associated with above mentioned pathologies and delayed wound healing of ulcers.

Keywords: Heparin Binding Epidermal Growth Factors, Endometriosis, Heart Pathologies, Rheumatoid Arthritis, Metastatic, Hormone Resistant Cancer.

Out of all Aurums, according to Hale, Aurum Muriaticum Natronatum is the most active of all the preparations of gold and possess more Cancerous Diathesis.

Homeopathic Indications

1. Nervous, Hysterical Women who are sensitive to pain, which drives them to despair.
2. Boring Pain.
3. Warts on tongue.
4. Metastasis to Bones.
5. Syphilitic Background.
6. Vexation leads to Jaundice.
7. Hypertrophy of Uterus.
8. Hysterical Spasms; starts from abdomen with pulsations in Occiput.
9. Coldness in abdomen.
10. Suicidal Impulse.
11. Vexed, Irritable.
12. Dirty looking teeth, that get loose; receding gums.
13. Black Gums.
14. Induration of one part; softening of another part.
15. Cancer of Breast with Fibroid Uterus.
16. Right Ovarian Dropsy with Uterine Fibroids.
17. Ovary+ Uterus+ Breast.
18. BRCA mutations and Ovary and Breast Cancer Syndrome.

3. Baryta Salts

Though Materia Medica and Repertory is full of indications of Baryta salts for Breast Cancer, no findings from latest chemical research confirms the carcinogenic property of Barium.

Barium is obtained from mineral ore, Baryte. Molecular structure of Radium and Barium are so similar that most of the times, substitution of Barium is done by Radium, or they may co-exist simultaneously in form of Radiobarite as in the ore of Radium, Pitchblende.

It might be the source from which the mother solution was made, if Radium would have been present in it as traces, the Cancer indications need to be attributed to the presence of Radium, and not the Barium.

At that time, no sophisticated techniques were developed to separate Radium from Barium or find traces of impurities.

Radium is a proven carcinogen possessing an ability to produce cancer, thus can cure cancer as well.

One may opt to use salts of Radium when indications of Baryta group is seen along with Cancer.

* Dr Grimmer has indicated Baryta Iodatum for Cancer after Injury to Breast.

4. Bromium

Bromine is a halogen from the fourth row of periodic table, occupying a place next to Arsenic and is also a hazardous, corrosive element, responsible for 30% depletion of ozone layer and has led to serious health problems in humans exposed to it. Bromine is extracted from sea water.

It is used in **Bread/fast foods**, purple dyes, hot tubs, nasal sprays, **citrus-flavored sodas**, fire retardant, electronics, carpets & upholstery, **pesticides,** photography, **pharmaceuticals** (mainly sedative, anticonvulsant), as fumigant, etc.

Health hazards due to Bromine include cough, asthma, lung disease, damage to kidney and liver, neurotoxic effect on the brain resulting in somnolence, psychosis, seizures, delirium and damage to DNA material. It is also a Carcinogen.

It equally competes with Iodine, depleting it from the body by binding itself with Iodine receptors which gives rise to **Hypothyroidism** and such Iodine deficiency also makes the breast prone to **Fibrocystic Disease** especially in young, perimenopausal woman finally resulting in **Estrogen Positive Breast Cancer.**

Keywords: Neurotoxicity; Lung Disease; Hypothyroidism; Fibrocystic Breast Disease; Psychosis; Perimenopausal Women; Estrogen Positive Breast Cancer

Homeopathic Indications

1. Blond type, Face grey, earthy, old-looking.

2. Inconsolable, sad, depressed during Cancer.

3. Extreme aversion to company and work.

4. Staring in one direction without saying anything.

5. Delusion someone else walks behind her.

6. Delusion death, coffin, ghost, spirits, seeing dead persons, funeral.

7. Sudden suffocation swallowing on.

8. Nosebleed accompanies many complaints; vicarious menses, from ears and nose.

9. Coldness in back while sitting.

10. Difficult Respiration during Menstruation.

11. Sadness, Melancholy, Dejection, Despondency, Gloom specially before and during menses

12. MENSES: DURING: EYES: FEEL AS IF THEY WOULD DROP OUT WHILE STOOPING.

13. Physometra.

14. Headache after drinking milk.

15. Affects the glands like thyroid, testis, maxillary and parotid.

16. WORSE, from evening, until midnight, and when sitting in warm room; warm damp weather; when at rest and lying left side.

17. BETTER, from any motion; exercise; at sea; Shaving.

18. Tendency to infiltrate glands, become hard but seldom suppurates.

19. Tumor in Breast, with stitching pains; worse on left side; from breast to axilla (Asterias Rubens).

20. Sharp, shooting pain in breast, < by pressure (rev. of Bryonia)

21. Stitches below mammae.

22. Breast cancer; nose bleed accompanies.

23. Tendency to metastasize to lungs.

5. Cadmium Metallicum

Cadmium is a transition metal from row 5, next to Silver; belonging to column 12, between Zinc and mercury.

Cadmium is a Teratogen, a Carcinogen and produces various health hazards.

Commercially, Cd is used in television screens, lasers, batteries, paint pigments, cosmetics, galvanizing steel, and also acts as a barrier in nuclear fission.

It is a proven Carcinogen. Tobacco plant absorbs large quantities of Cadmium from the soil and Smoking is one of the main routes of its contamination, others being a sea organism, like Asterias Rubens, , and occupational exposure.

The toxicity produces a typical yellow ring at the base of teeth with caries.

Cadmium induces tissue injury by creating oxidative stress, epigenetic changes in DNA expression. It causes apoptosis of neutrons impairing learning capacity, memory and attentiveness. It may also destroy hearing and olfactory faculties.

It replaces Zn and Mg from the body and hinders their physiological function.

Cadmium may also impair Vitamin D metabolism in the kidney, causes severe pain from osteomalacia with osteoporosis, renal tubular dysfunction, anemia affecting spleen, and calcium malabsorption.

It also works on CVS and Kidney together and produces Insulin Resistant Diabetes Mellitus and Hypertension.[48]

Being an endocrine disrupter, it disturbs functions of Pituitary. Cadmium is a strong Metaloestrogen and binds to Alpha Estrogen receptors of body producing Estrogen Positive Breast cancer.[49]

It is also linked with Lung, Kidney, Pancreatic and Non-Hodgkin's Lymphoma.

Keywords: Carcinogen, Smoking, Yellow ring at base of teeth, Kidney, Bone Pains, Spleen, Metaloestrogen, Estrogen Positive Breast Cancer

Homeopathic Indications

1. According to Dr Grimmer, "what Sulphur is to Psora, Cadmium is to Cancer". Cadmium salts were extensively used during cancer treatment with noteworthy results.

2. Pathologies move towards death.

3. Highly chilly, feels chilly even near the stove (Cad Sulph.).

4. Craves water but it causes goose pimple to appear Cad. Sulph.).

5. Debility of Arsenic + Motion Aversion to like Bryonia+ Neurological symptoms like Zincum (Cad. Sulph.).

6. Irritative action of alumina toxin resulting from aluminum cooking utensils.

7. Vertigo while looking at moving pictures accompanied with sensation of something taking the breath away, objects recede and return.

8. Paralysis when Causticum Fails.

9. Sleeps with eyes open.

10. Impulsive irritability, up to the verge of insanity in its violence, alternating with a deep depression of the mind.

11. Loathing of life, hopeless and apathetic, all joy is gone.

12. Unable to concentrate, saying and doing the wrong things such as putting salt in her tea instead of sugar.

13. Vivid, unhappy dreams of sickness, causing worry after awakening.

14. Averse to people, certain kinds of music; noise.

15. Odors and unpleasant things produce nausea, even when thinking of them.

16. State of indifference, desire to be alone, improved by appearance of a skin eruption.

17. Dreams of running without reaching anywhere.

18. Depressive psychosis with fear of cancer.

19. Amelioration from eating, pressure, cold application, bending double, pressure appearance of an eruption.

20. Aggravation in the morning; from waking either daytime or night; movement; mental effort.

21. Frequent urination, discoloring the vessel brownish or deep lemon color, very hard to wash off the vessel.

6. Calcarea Salts

Calcarea Carbonicum and other salts are well-known remedies for lymphatic constitution and are well reputed for their anti-cancer diathesis.

Scientists have recently discovered Nanoparticles of Calcium changing acidic pH of blood to alkaline, arresting growth of malignant cells. According to Otto Warburg, a Nobel Laurette, cancer cells require acidic medium to grow as they cannot survive in alkaline medium.

Calcarea Carb has characteristic symptom of sourness of system marked by acidity, and sour smelling body and discharges.

Homeopathic indications

Calcarea Flourica

1. When all the remedies fail, Calc. flour helps.
2. When the patient has stony-hard Breast Tumors with metastasis to bones.
3. Induration and threatening suppuration.
4. A remedy for varicose and enlarged veins, and also malnutrition of bones.

Calcarea Phosphorica

1. Suits to thin individuals, with anemic and dark complexion, with dark hair and eyes.
2. Always wants to go somewhere.
3. Mentally peevish, forgetful after grief and vexation.
4. Complaints aggravate when thinking about them.
5. Hunger at 4 p.m.
6. Crawling and coldness.
7. Non-union of bones and also promotes callous.
8. Spine weak, disposed to curvatures, especially to left.
9. Weak neck with inability to support head.
10. Rheumatic pain from draught of air with stiffness and dullness of head.
11. Stiffness and pain with cold, numb feeling < change of weather.
12. Pain in sacroiliac symphysis as if broken.
13. Pains in joints and bones.
14. In females, there is increased sexual desire before menses and during lactation.

15. Child refuses breast; milk tastes salty.
16. A remedy for breast cancer metastasis to bones.
17. Useful in case of tumor in left mammae of males, which is painful on pressure.

7. Carbons'

Carbon compounds possess immense therapeutic applications in cancer treatment, especially for Breast Cancer.

Homeopathic Indications
Carbolic Acid

1. Belladonna-like pain+ Malignant ulcer+ Offensiveness.
2. Terrible pain, comes suddenly; lasts for a short time and disappears suddenly.
3. Breast cancer; of left breast (Bromium, Asterias).
4. Longing for whiskey and tobacco.
5. When a burn tends to ulcerate (after effects of radiation).
6. Constipation with horribly offensive breath.
7. Green Leucorrhoea (Secale Cornutum).
8. Involuntary Discharges.
9. Last stage of Cancer.

Graphites

1. Patients who are stout, of fair complexion, with tendency to skin affections and constipation.
2. Fat, chilly and costive with delayed menstrual history.
3. Mammae Cancer from old cicatrices, which has remained after repeated abscesses.

Carbo Animalis

1. Bone metastasis with Cancer of breast and cachexia in later stages.

2. Tumors with debility and slowness.
3. Darting in breast; painful indurations in breast especially in right breast.
4. Keynote: Cancer with mental state of Natrum muriaticum.
5. Patient avoids company and has a desire to be alone, is sad and depressed.
6. Aversion to meat, milk and fats.
7. Cannot tolerate heat or cold.
8. Coldness of extremities.
9. Aggravation from salt.
10. Abdomen pain in acute situations > by flatus and stools.
11. Drawing cramping pain in calf during walking.
12. Suffocation at night on closing eyes.

8. Fluorine

Fluorine is the most electronegative element, hence it is rarely found alone. This extraordinary stability has made it an excellent carrier, and is therefore, extensively used in almost 20% of pharmaceuticals and 30% of agricultural products, though it has no biological function. Rather it is a debated carcinogen with so many health hazards. Endemic Fluorosis is one of the major health concerns crippling millions of people worldwide every year.

In some countries, it is added to drinking water and also used in toothpaste globally for its supposed ability to prevent dental caries. Besides drinking water, medicines like Dexamethasone, Fluoxetine, Statins, etc., food, occupational exposure, extensive use in agriculture, **Tea Drinking** are also responsible for Systemic Fluorosis.

Fluorine is extremely toxic and corrosive substance and has an extraordinary appetite to bind to Calcium Ions. Once it enters the system, it seeks calcium forming Calcium Fluoride crystals in joints and bones producing severe pain, arthritis, osteoporosis and enlarged joints causing difficulty in movements. It also affects Parathyroid gland by increasing serum calcium level, thus affecting heart function, thyroid gland and causing collagen disorders, atherosclerosis, hypertension, diabetes mellitus, obesity, rupture of ligaments and other health hazards.[50]

Fluorine has the property of ossifying the Pineal gland, thus affecting Pituitary and endocrine system as well. Pineal gland ossification leads to reduced Melatonin production affecting Circadian Rhythm, early onset of Puberty and increased hormone positive breast cancer risks. Fluorine is also linked with Osteosarcoma, Lymphoma and other cancers.[51]

Keywords: Fluorosis; Binding Calcium; Parathyroid Gland; Thyroid Gland, Pituitary Gland, Pineal Gland, Hormone Positive Breast Cancer; Osteosarcoma

Homeopathic Indications

1. Premature Aging.
2. Indifference towards to loved ones; animated to strangers.
3. Inability to realize responsibilities.
4. Buoyancy.
5. Involuntary Sighing.
6. Increased ability to exercise without fatigue (Coca), tolerance to extreme of temperature.
7. Complete Forgetfulness.
8. APPREHENSION: DANGER: AS IF MENACED BY: WITHOUT FEAR.
9. Bloated Glabella.
10. Large patches of alopecia; new hair dry and breaks off; must comb of the hair often, it mats so at the end baldness.
11. Rapid Caries of Teeth.
12. Varicosities.

13. Hemangioma.
14. Caries and Necrosis, especially for long bones.
15. Fistula.
16. Exostosis.
17. Coccygodynia.
18. Sudden dropsical swelling with craving for refreshing drinks.
19. Complete Paralysis.
20. Indurated Ulcers with Red Edges.
21. Liver Disorders as a consequence of alcoholic drinks.
22. Metrorrhagia with dyspnea.
23. Mouth Ulcers During Menses.
24. MAMMAE: INFLAMMATION: CHRONIC, WITH PAIN.
25. MAMMAE: ITCHING: LEFT, ON. (0>1>0)
26. Nipples: Cracked, Red, Itching.
27. Last stage of Breast Cancer, often used with Tarentula Cubensis.
28. Useful for Palliation.

9. Iodine

Iodine is the last halogen from 5th row.

Iodine compounds are used as catalyst, animal feed supplements, stabilizers, dyes, colorants and pigments, pharmaceuticals, for sanitation and photography as they are highly antimicrobial and antiviral in action.

Iodine is an essential nutrient for body and the heaviest element a human requires for the normal functioning of Thyroid Gland, Breast Development and Estrogen Balance.

Deficiency of Iodine leads to impaired function of Thyroid gland, Goiter, Obesity, Decreased Metabolism, Retardation of Intellectual Faculties, Fibrocystic Breast Disease and also makes one prone to Breast Cancer. Food sources rich in natural Iodine like sea weed are found to be associated with prevention of Breast Cancer. Supplementation of Molecular Iodine is recommended in patients suffering from Breast Cancer for a better outcome of treatment by nutritionists.[52]

There are three kinds of Estrogen, namely Estrone, Estradiol and Estriole. They are controlled by Iodine.

Estrone and Estradiol are related with PMS, Breast tenderness, Obesity and also act as Carcinogen. Their secretion is diminished by Iodine while, while **Estriole,** an anti-Estradiol, produced by adipose tissue and not by ovary, are helpful in weight reduction, its secretion is stimulated by Iodine.

Its concentration rises during pregnancy as it helps in the development of fetal organs.

Estriole is also used in Hormone Replacement Therapy.

Excess of Iodine and Estriole leads to weight reduction; shrinkage of mammary glands, hyperthyroidism and are also related with increased incidence of Thyroid and Breast cancer.[53]

Keywords: Breast Health; Weight Management; Anti Estradiol; Estriole; Thyroid; Breast and Thyroid Cancer

Homeopathic Indications

1. Persons of scrofulous diathesis, with dark or black hair and eyes.
2. Tearful and sad; shuns persons; anxious, apprehensive, restless, agitated; must move about; irresistible impulse to run; feels she will fall if she walks; cross, irritable, impulse to murder; excessive mental excitement; averse to any type of intellectual labor.
3. Fixed ideas.
4. Affected by the moon's changes.

5. Heart palpates like lightning; effects of amorousness and disappointed love.

6. Ravenous hunger; eats freely and well, yet loses flesh all the time.

7. Atrophy and emaciation till reduced to the state of a skeleton (with good appetite).

8. Absence of appetite is also among the effects of Iod., and either condition may indicate it.

9. Feels ameliorated while eating or after eating, when stomach is full.

10. Salty taste.

11. Salivary glands and pancreas are affected.

12. Aggravation: Warmth; wrapping up the head (reverse of, Hep., Psor.).

13. Great weakness and loss of breath on going upstairs (Calc.); during the menses (Alum, Carbo an., Coc.); even speaking excites perspiration.

14. Nocturnal sweat, pulse quick, small, and hard.

15. Sleeplessness.

16. Distortion of the bones.

17. Hypertrophy and induration of glandular tissue like thyroid, mammae, ovaries, testes, uterus, prostate of other glands, breasts may dwindle and become flabby.

18. Hard goiter, in dark - haired persons (light – haired persons, Brom.).

19. Constipation ameliorated by drinking cold milk.

20. Edematous swelling, even of the whole body.

21. Leucorrhea: yellow, acrid, corrosive, staining and corroding the linen.

22. Complete loss of sexual power, atrophy of ovaries and mammae, with sterility, offensive sweating of genitals.

23. Dwindling and falling away of the mammae.

24. MENSES: DURING: MAMMAE: DARTING.
25. Menses: during: mammae: dwindling.
26. Lactation: milk: flow, involuntary.
27. LACTATION: MILK: PROFUSE, TOO: THIN, WATERY.
28. Lactation: milk: suppressed.
29. Mammae: atrophy.
30. MAMMAE: ATROPHY: DROPSY, OVARIAN.
31. Mammae: induration: bluish red nodosities, size of a hazelnut, dry, black points at tips.
32. Mammae: relaxed.
33. Mammae: sensitive: hyperesthesia.
34. Mammae: sharp pain: metritis, in.
35. Mammae: sharp pain: womb, in cancer of.

10. Mercury and its salts

Mercury comes under world's top ten most hazardous elements and is also one of the most probable carcinogens.

Homeopathic Materia Medica is full of indications for Mercury and its salts for various cancerous states proving their carcinogenicity. Mercury is the king of the anti-miasmatic remedies against Syphilis.

Mercury like Lead is also environmental pollutant and contaminates air, water and soil. One of the food chains of mercury is Fish. Other sources include its use in dental amalgam and as a preservative in vaccines.

Methylmercury is most poisonous of all mercury salts, due to its organic and biotic origin, and is produced by action of bacteria on mercury.

Mercury and Methylmercury are **Metaloestrogen**[54] which denotes that they mimic estrogen (other such metals are Cadmium, Aluminum, Plumbum, Nickel, Arsenic, Antimony and Cobalt) and bind to Alfa Receptors of Estrogen, producing Estrogen positive Breast Cancer, especially in post-menopausal women.

A study[55] has found methylmercury effective against breast cancer lines.

Keywords: Pollutant; Toxic; Metaloestrogen; Estrogen Positive Breast Cancer; Post-menopausal Women

Homeopathic Indications

Mercurius Iodatum Flavus

1. Mammary tumors with the tendency to warm perspiration and gastric disturbances.
2. Thickly coated tongue; yellow at the base.
3. The tip and edges may be red and take imprints of teeth.
4. Throat affections.
5. Greatly swollen glands.
6. Worse on right side.
7. Lacunar tonsillitis, when only superficial part of tonsil is involved.
8. Cheesy exudates with offensive breath.
9. Constant inclination to swallow.
10. Nausea at the sight or odor of food.
11. Thirst for sour drinks.
12. Worse on right tonsil with much tenacious mucus.

Mercurius Bin Kali Iodatum

1. Leading remedy for Bone Metastasis.
2. Tumors of bones with Hodgkin's Lymphoma.
3. Tubercular history.
4. Mind symptoms are similar to Staphysagria.

11. Platina

Platinum is a highly valuable, rare, noble metal.

Platina is well indicated in literature for Ovary, Breast and Brain Cancer.

In the chemical medicines also, Platinum based compounds like Cisplatin, Carboplatin and Oxaliplatin, are one of the most important chemotherapeutic agents which work by damaging crosslinks between DNA strands, producing apoptosis.

They are found to be more effective *for BRCA mutation and Triple Negative Kind of Breast Cancers.* All three of them are effective for cancer but are equally oncogenic and have lots of side effects.

Based on the Law of Similars, they can be employed in potentized form to treat Cancer with symptoms of Platina and their relative side effects.

These Compounds are discussed in the chapter of synthetic sources.

Homeopathic Indications

1. Dark-haired females.
2. Face changes color frequently.
3. Strong tendency to Paralysis, Anesthesia.
4. Hysterical spasms; at day break.
5. Great inclination to violent, almost spasmodic, yawning.
6. Changing moods, sad and gay alternately, laughs and cries by turns.
7. Irresistible impulse to kill.
8. Self-exaltation; CONTEMPT FOR OTHERS. Arrogant, proud.
9. Nymphomania. Excessive sexual development; vaginismus.

10. Abnormal sexual appetite and melancholia.

11. Affections caused by fright, by vexation, or by a fit of passion.

12. Weary of everything. Everything seems changed.

13. Mental troubles associated with suppressed menses.

14. Pains increase and decrease gradually. (STANNUM)

15. Physical symptoms disappear as mental symptoms develop.

16. Sensitiveness of parts.

17. COLDNESS, CREEPING, AND NUMBNESS.

18. Menstruation, when the discharge is very abundant, thick and black like tar, and is very exhausting, Spasms and screaming at every menstrual period.

19. Leucorrhoea, like white of eggs, flowing chiefly after urinating, rising from a seat, only during day.

20. Pruritus vulvae.

21. Ovaritis with sterility.

22. Postpartum: vulva, sensitive, cannot bear touch of napkin.

23. Mammae: shooting: violent, two or three times a day, from side along lower portion of left, with nausea and giddiness.

12. Plumbum

Lead is an environmental pollutant, listed under probable carcinogens and gets released in the environment via petrol fumes, paints and multiple other sources.

It is linked to lung, kidney and brain cancers.

It is stored in the bones and gets released during process of bone demineralization during the menopause. Such endogenous increased level of Plumbum is nephrotoxic and is associated with Hypertension.[56]

A study in Nigeria has found increased level of Plumbum and decreased levels of Selenium and Iodine in women of postmenopausal age with infiltrating Breast Duct Carcinoma than normal women of same age, indicating the increased presence of Plumbum in the body associated with the given pathology.[57]

It replaces Selenium, a cancer protective element in the body, and binds with cancer preventive Iodine, thus can alter thyroid functions causing malignancy or hastening its process.

Plumbum iodatum is found to disrupt reproductive system and alter hormonal levels as well.

Keywords: Plumbism; Kidney; Osteoporosis; Hypertension; Thyroid; Post-menopausal Women; Hormone Positive; Infiltrating Ductal Breast Cancer

Homeopathic Indications

1. Blue line across the gums.
2. Progressive Emaciation.
3. Constipation.
4. Weakness.
5. Atherosclerosis.
6. Hypertension.
7. Paralysis with muscular atrophy, arteriosclerosis, sclerous degeneration of the marrow.
8. Enlarged glands and chronic enlargement of the spleen.
9. Pellagra.
10. Amenorrhea from atrophy of the ovaries.
11. Indurations of great hardness and associated with a very dry skin.
12. Indurations of mammary glands, especially when a tendency to become inflamed appears; sore and painful.

Chapter 7

Nosodes

Nosodes are the medicines prepared from potentized diseased tissue or diseased product.

A Nosode is prescribed in the following conditions:

1. When it is indicated as a Constitutional Remedy after case taking and matches the symptom totality on the basis of Individuality.
2. As an Intercurrent Remedy, when well selected remedies fail due to a miasmatic blockage.
3. When there is a Positive Family History of Cancer in the patient, in the beginning or during the treatment.
4. To Strengthen the Constitution in order to respond to the homeopathic remedy with a Past History of Cancer or Premalignant lesion.
5. To Prevent the Occurrence or Relapse of Cancer in patients with past or family history of cancer.
6. To complete the cure.

The important Cancer Nosodes include:

1. Carcinosinum
2. Scirrhinum

Carcinosinum

1. Carcinosin is made up from cancerous breast tissues.

2. Adapted to persons with brownish, café-au-lait complexion.

3. Adapted to blue, sclerotic individuals with numerous moles, warts, birth mark anywhere in the body.

4. It is useful when the indicated remedy partially improves or fails to cure or only ameliorates temporarily .

5. H/o recurrent attack of bronchitis, pneumonia, whooping cough, measles, chicken pox, tonsillitis, diphtheria or any infectious diseases etc. or absence of any infectious diseases in childhood.

6. H/o Insomnia in childhood.

7. Family history of cancer, tuberculosis, diabetes, pernicious anemia, syphilis.

8. Craving, aversion, or intolerance of salt, sweet, meat, egg, milk, fat and fruit or all of these.

9. Position of patient in sleep is knee-elbow position, curling up like a dog.

10. Better or worse in sea air.

11. Tendency to insomnia.

12. Very much fastidious; wants everything neat and clean.

13. Enjoys rainy season.

14. Marked sensitivity to rhythm, love or dancing or sensitivity of music.

15. Wants to travel.

16. Extremely sensitive to reprimands with suppressed emotions like Staphysagria and Ignatia.

Scirrhinum

1. It is alike to Carcinosinum; but the tumor itself is harder.
2. This is a valuable intercurrent remedy to be given during the course of constitutional treatment, enhancing and complementing the action of indicated remedies. (Dr Grimmer)
3. Present with stomach symptoms similar to Sulphur like "hollow sensation at the umbilicus and a history of worms."
4. Tremendous sinking at the naval region.
5. < from 5 p.m. to 6 p.m.
6. Swollen sensation in abdomen.
7. H/o Expulsion of pinworms.
8. Suicidal disposition or hereditary.
9. Lancinating pain of Cancer.
10. Hemorrhages and varicosities of legs and feet, with purple points.

Chapter 8

Sarcodes

Sarcodes are defined as the remedies prepared from healthy tissues, glands or organs.

Sarcodes can be prescribed in the following two ways:

1. **As a supplement in crude form**

   Extract form or low potency like 1X, 3X, etc of a Nosode is usually recommended in cases of severe Hypofunction or after surgical removal/injury/radiation of a secretory gland or organ. This is done as a measure to meet the requirements of the deficiency mainly caused due to unnatural events or due to grave pathologies with structural damage of an important organ or gland.

   For example, Thyroidinum in X potency when thyroid gland is hypofunctioning after radiation cycles in the throat area and this deficiency is evident by clinical signs and symptoms.

   Sometimes, ovarian extracts are required after surgical removal of ovaries if a patient shows disturbances afterwards due to lack of Estrogen.

2. **As a Homeopathic Remedy in Potentized Form**

   Potentized remedy is given when it is indicated as a constitutional remedy on the basis of symptom similarity.

   When the well-selected remedies fail and role of an organ, gland or tissues seems central to the pathology presented, potentized form is useful.

It can also be given when there is paucity of characteristic symptoms or only few symptoms are present due to exaggerated, or absence or malfunctioning of a physiological process.

Also as an intercurrent remedy during the treatment of diseases with deep structural changes to boost the functioning of a debilitated organ or gland.

Potentized remedy helps to remove the obstacles to cure when presenting symptoms occur because of disruption of hormonal cycle due to lifestyle, use of synthetic hormones or acute emotions which lead to endocrinal crisis or imbalance.

Endocrine Glands involved in Breast Carcinogenesis include:

1. Pineal Gland
2. Hypothalamus
3. Pituitary
4. Thymus
5. Mammary Gland
6. Thyroid
7. Adrenaline
8. Ovaries

1. Pineal Gland

Pineal gland is a small endocrine gland present inside the brain of most vertebrates. It produces melatonin, a serotonin-derived hormone, *which modulates sleep patterns in both circadian and seasonal cycles.*

It is a gland of endocrinal and spiritual significance and controls functions of all the other endocrinal glands of body. It is related to the "third eye", an eye which gives inner enlightenment and spiritual awakening.

This gland influences the pituitary gland's secretion of the sex hormones, follicle-stimulating hormone (FSH), and luteinizing hormone (LH).

Pineal-derived melatonin mediates its action on the bone cells through MT2 receptors.

Its effect on Breast:

Melatonin inhibits the ovarian glands from increasing in size, hence limiting the production of hormones like estrogen, progesterone, FSH and LH, which increase the rate of cellular growth in the breast, thus leading to greater chances of genetic error and breast cancer.

Some studies have also found that women with lower levels of melatonin, such as those who work in night shift or sleep for few hours, have a higher risk of developing breast cancer.

Homeopathic Indications

1. Bad Effects of disruption of natural biological rhythm or Circadian rhythm.
2. Effects of Late Night Watching and being in front of blue lights of mobile/TV till late night.
3. People who works in night shifts.
4. History of working in artificial lights for prolonged time.
5. Interruption of natural menstrual cycle through artificial hormones.
6. Precocious Sexual Development and Maturity.
7. Abnormal amount of fat.
8. Progressive Muscular Dystrophy.
9. Tumor with persistent headache.

2. Pituitary Gland

Growth hormone

The major **role** *of* **growth hormone** *in stimulating body* **growth** *is to stimulate the liver and other tissues to secrete IGF-I.*

IGF-I stimulates proliferation of chondrocytes (cartilage cells), resulting in bone **growth**.

It also mediates body metabolism releasing energy.

Its effect on Breast:

Growth hormone plays a significant role in the development, progression, and metastasis of Breast Cancer by influencing tumor angiogenesis, stemness, and chemoresistance.

Follicle Stimulating Hormone and Luteinizing Hormone:

FSH and LH *are hormones essential* for pubertal development and functioning of ovaries. In women, these hormones stimulate the growth of ovarian follicles in the ovary before the release of an egg from one follicle at ovulation. It also increases estradiol production.

Its effect on Breast:

FSH and LH receptors and the related signaling intermediates are necessary for the actions of gonadotrophins on cytoskeletal rearrangement, migration and invasion of the cells of Breast Cancer.

Homeopathic Indications of Folliculinum

(Ref: Dr Julian's Materia Medica)

1.   Extreme instability, with anguish, worse at nightfall.

2. Alternation of excitability and depression, worse before menses.

3. Sexual hyper-excitability.

4. Fixed ideas, of a sexual nature.

5. Hypersensitive to heat, noise and contact.

6. Congestive headache, either with redness of the face, or with pallor, along with the sensation of chilliness at the extremities.

7. Pre-menstrual migraines.

8. Congestive mastitis.

9. Obesity, with water and fat retention.

10. Fibroma.

11. Sterility.

12. Physiological complaints in women during menstruation.

13. Menopausal complaints.

14. Chronic B. Coli infections.

15. Juvenile acne in both sexes.

16. Chapping eczema.

17. Acne on the face, and seborrhoea of the nostrils.

18. Dry eczema, worse during ovulation, before menses.

19. Alopecia in women.

20. Swelling, edema of the conjunctival tissue and nucleus having cellulitis.

21. Weight gain, without excessive eating, worse before menses or during ovulation.

22. Recurring cystitis in women.

23. Feminizing tumours of the ovary, persistent follicle, follicular cysts.

24. Allergy to Estrogen, Conditions of hypersensitivity.

25. Dysmenorrhea. Prolonged intervals between menses. Pre-menstrual leucorrhea.

26. Vulvar pruritus, worse before menses.

27. Loss of blood during ovulation.
28. Menses prolonged, blood bright red, with clotting.
29. Yellow or brownish discharge sometimes blood streaked, between menses, especially during ovulation.
30. Fibroid Uterus, with metrorrhagia.
31. Congestion, pre-menstrual pains.
32. Breasts enormously swollen, cannot bear being constricted or touched.
33. The pain ameliorates or disappears with menses.
34. <before menses, during ovulation, from heat and from resting.
35. >After the third day of menses, with movement, fresh air.

3. Prolactin

Prolactin is originally named for its function, i.e. *to promote milk production (lactation)*.

It is also associated with breast development, especially stromal part of breast.

Its effect on Breast:

A positive association prevails between plasma prolactin levels and the risk of Breast Cancer among the postmenopausal patients suffering from ER$^+$/PR$^+$ *or* in-situ *and invasive carcinoma.*

Homeopathic Indications of Pituitarinum:

1. Phosphor-fluoric types, tubercular poisoning, or syphilitic, with obsessional or depressive psychopathic complaints.
2. Weeping, the patient cries involuntarily and even without noticing.
3. Obsessive ideas linked to the urogenital area.
4. Memory: difficulty or inability to fix attention.

5. Weary of life.

6. Nocturnal anxiety.

7. Due to its action on the uterus and mammary glands, it is one of the sheer-anchors in delayed puberty and stunted growth with amenorrhea and atrophy of breasts, due to endocrine imbalance.

8. Obstinate cases of spasmodic dysmenorrhea.

9. High blood pressure, chronic nephritis.

10. Polyuria, at times, with glycosuria.

11. Abnormal deposits of fat, loss of hair, of sexual power, and atrophy of the ovaries.

12. Fat deposition, particularly in the lower abdomen, hairs turned grey.

13. Congestive headache associated with menses.

14. Pigmentation disorders, and loss of hair.

15. Menses late: cycle longer than 30 days.

16. Menses, with pain just before, and during the day.

17. Atrophy of the mammary glands: growth of hair on chest.

18. Amenorrhoea, with mammary atrophy.

19. Mammary hypertrophy.

4. Thyroid Gland

Thyroid hormones act on nearly every cell in the body to increase the basal metabolic rate, and also affect protein synthesis, help regulate long bone growth (synergy with growth hormone) and neural maturation, and increase the body's sensitivity to catecholamines (such as adrenaline) by permissiveness.

Its effect on Breast:

Breast and thyroid cancers are two malignancies with highest incidence in women.

Women with thyroid cancer are at increased risk for subsequent Breast Cancer; and vice-versa, suggestive of a common etiology.

Hypothyroidism is generally associated with postmenopausal Breast Cancer while hyperthyroidism is with premenopausal Breast Cancer.

Breast Cancer is a hormone dependent malignancy. Moreover, hormonal therapy also may disrupt the Thyroid Functions.

As already stated under Iodum that thyroid and Breast Cancer are linked to each other and Iodine plays a vital role in Breast development and Estrogen Balance.

In order to finetune the imbalanced Thyroid gland; as a Sarcode and as an Individual Constitutional Remedy; Thyroidinum is commonly used.

Homeopathic Indications of Thyroidinum

1. Easy tiredness, coma, extreme chilliness, tremors, low metabolism.
2. Allergies+ Calcarea-like+ Vasomotor affections.
3. Allergies of different kinds.
4. Suspicious.
5. Delusion Persecuted.
6. Idiocy; Arrested development like Baryta Carb.
7. < by least contradiction.
8. Fearful nightmares.
9. Wants to lie down, does not want to do anything with anyone.
10. Malice> lying on bed.
11. Rests in recumbent position, extreme breathlessness with lividity.
12. Fat, perspiring, chilly.

13. Falling of hair.

14. Perspiration on palms.

15. Brown colored spots.

16. Excessive appetite.

17. Desire for sweets and thirst for cold water.

18. Rolling flatulence with gurgling, loose, gassy stools.

19. Polyuria especially in Diabetes.

20. Vasodilatation, Increased blood pressure.

21. Puerperal convulsion, insanity.

22. < During Pregnancy.

23. History of use of Oral Contraceptive pills.

24. Mammary Tumors; Agalactia; Uterine Fibroids.

25. Clinically indicated in 2X potency for fibroid tumors of breast.

5. Adrenal gland

Adrenalin is called Stress/ fight / flight hormone.

Key actions of adrenaline include increasing the heart rate, increasing blood pressure, expanding the air passages of the lungs, enlarging the pupil in the eye, redistributing blood to the muscles and altering the body's metabolism, so as to maximize blood glucose levels (primarily for the brain) which happens during acute threat, for example when a wild animal chase a person in darkness.

Chronic stress and unresolved anxieties keeps circulating Adrenaline levels elevated to cope with the perceived threat with health consequences including Breast Cancer.

It feeds the Cancer Stem Cells resulting in treatment resistant and relapsing cancers.

Homeopathic Indications

1. Cowardly, despondent, nervous, distracted, averse to mental labor.

2. Despondent and nervous; lack of interest in anything; no ambition; disinclination for mental work; absence of "grit."

3. Aversion to mental work, cannot concentrate thoughts.

4. Doubtful recovery of; medicine is useless.

5. Desire to remain on bed, morose, indifferent.

6. Bronzed skin, rapid pulse, loss of strength and wasting.

7. Vertigo, turning on right side ameliorates.

8. Lack of vital heat, cold food cold water.

9. The face flushed, but not red.

10. Tongue coated white, red edge and tip.

11. Swallowing impossible; constriction of esophagus.

12. Sudden spluttering diarrhea; all over in a minute, followed with burning in anus.

13. Obstinate constipation.

14. Hematuria.

15. Cancer of uterus and rectum and mammae.

16. Cancer patient with adrenal disturbance.

6. Ovaries

The ovaries are active from puberty to menopause, during which they perform the functions of ovulation and also produce substances that are necessary in the maintaining of certain female characteristics.

If young girls are castrated, the pelvis does not show a normal development, the voice is lower, more or less hair develops on the face, the legs are longer. The castrated female takes on the male type.

The earlier a girl menstruates, the shorter the legs, the later it appears, the longer the legs.

Early sexual development in the girl is the result of rapid functional development of the ovaries or hypofunction of the pineal gland.

Ovarian Hormones are associated with breast development and are associated with 70-80% of all Breast Cancers.

Oophorinum is made up from healthy ovaries.

Homeopathic Indications

1. Female of today's generation.
2. Early menopausal symptom like restlessness and irritability.
3. Sweating like hot flushes, osteoarthritic changes and hairy growth on face.
4. Severe Climacteric Flushing when Lachesis and other remedies have failed.
5. Obesity.
6. Depression.
7. Low blood pressure.
8. Chilly.
9. History of over the counter usage of Oral Contraceptive Pills.
10. Hysteria ad other neurotic manifestation.
11. Profuse uterine hemorrhage.
12. Uterine fibroid.
13. H/o PCOD.
14. Physical debility, mental depression and melancholia.
15. Increased sexual desire.

7. Estrogen

Estrogen forms unique relationships with other hormones in the breast, which are responsible for:

1.   the growth of the breasts during adolescence.

2. the pigmentation of the nipples
3. stopping the flow of milk when an infant is no longer breast-feeding.
4. It acts through Estrogen Receptors present in the cells.
5. It has wide and complex biological in role affecting multiple organs and system including psyche.

Breast Cancer is a Hormonal Event as more than 70% of breast cancers are Hormone Positive; mainly Estrogen Positive.

Estrogen, whose excess, deficiency or disturbance plays a central role in Breast Carcinogenesis, is a Sarcode of utmost value.

Homeopathic Indications

It requires a detailed proving, though the indications based on Dr Sarkar's clinical experience are mentioned as follows:

1. Combination of Breast Modalities+ Liver derangement + Endometriosis.
2. Breast Cancer with severe migraine.
3. Fullness and tenderness of breast.
4. Endometriosis, endometrial cancer with history of oral contraceptive pills.
5. Breast cancer with gall bladder involvement.
6. Female offsprings of mothers who had Di-Ethyl Stilbestrol (DES) during first trimester.

Symptoms of Estradiol from Marsh' Clinical Drugs are:

1. Endocrine Pancreatitis.
2. Peripheral edema.
3. Abdominal cramping or bloating; anorexia (loss of appetite); nausea; diarrhea; vomiting.
4. Gallbladder obstruction; hepatitis.
5. Endometrial atrophy; increase in libido.

6. Menopausal symptoms; atrophic vaginitis.
7. Amenorrhea; breakthrough bleeding; heavier vaginal bleeding between regular menses; menorrhagia; spotting.
8. Breast pain or tenderness; enlargement of breasts.
9. Breast tumors; breast lumps; discharge from breast.

8. Progesterone

Progesterone prepares the inner lining of endometrium for conception, and also stimulates the growth of milk ducts in the breasts.

Its effect on Breast:

About 80% of all Breast Cancers are "ER-positive," i.e. the cancer cells grow in response to the hormone estrogen. About 65% of these are "PR-positive" which grow in response to another hormone, progesterone.

Homeopathic Indications

Mental Symptoms (Ref.: Dr Murphy's Lotus Materia Medica):

1. Loss of concentration. Foggy thinking.
2. Inability to make decisions.
3. Inability to handle even the smallest amount of stress.
4. Anxiety, irritability. Anger. Anti-social.
5. Panic attacks.
6. Very emotional, feeling overwhelmed. Mood changes.
7. Severe depression.
8. Feeling of despair and hopelessness.
9. Uncontrollable crying, immense sadness.
10. Suicidal depression. Psychotic.
11. Delusion, feels like they are in another's body.

Other Symptoms (Ref.: Dr Marsh's Clinical Drugs):

1. Secondary amenorrhea; functional uterine bleeding; endometriosis.

2. Mental depression; dizziness; drowsiness; headache; mood changes; nervousness; insomnia.

3. Hypotension; thromboembolism.

4. Adrenal suppression or insufficiency; Cushing's syndrome.

5. Amenorrhea; breakthrough menstrual bleeding; metromenorrhagia; menorrhagia; spotting; galactorrhea; ovarian enlargement; ovarian cyst formation; breast pain or tenderness; hot flushes.

6. Oedema; fatigue, unusual or rapid weight gain.

7. Abdominal pain or cramping; diarrhoea; nausea; vomiting.

8. Hyperglycemia.

9. Decrease in Libido.

10. Skin rash; acne; loss or gain of body, facial or scalp hair; melasma.

9. Testosterone

Testosterone plays an important role in females for their sex drive, bone mass and vaginal health.

Women with high testosterone levels, either due to disease or drug use, may experience a decrease in breast size.

Its effects on Breast:

Higher levels of androgens in the blood may be linked to an increased risk of Breast Cancer in women.

Homeopathic Indications

According to Dr Murphy in Nature Materia Medica and Dr Marsh's Clinical Drugs:

1. Crying; depersonalization; dysphoria; euphoria.
2. Mental depression; paranoia; quick to react or overreact emotionally; rapidly changing moods.
3. Headache; anxiety; insomnia.
4. Acne; alopecia; increase in pubic hair growth.
5. Symptoms of fatigue, malaise, loss of sex drive, and loss of muscle tissue.
6. Increased facial and body hair, oily skin, male pattern baldness, water retention, joint stiffness.
7. A deepened or hoarse voice.
8. Bleeding. Emaciation. Fatigue
9. Hypertension. Erythrocytosis; secondary polycythaemia; leukopenia.
10. Bladder irritability; urinary tract infection.
11. Cholestatic jaundice; hepatic necrosis; hepatocellular tumor; Pelosi's hepatis.
12. Hypercalcemia.
13. Growth of the clitoris, and menstrual irregularities.
14. Amenorrhoea; oligomenorrhea; virilism.
15. Decrease or increase in libido.
16. Cancer.

10. Thymus

The thymus plays a vital role in the training and development of T-lymphocytes or T-cells, an extremely important type of white blood cell. T-cells defend the body from potentially deadly pathogens such as bacteria, viruses, and fungi.

The stock of T-lymphocytes is built up in early life, so the function of the thymus is diminished in adults.

It is largely degenerated in elderly adults and is barely identifiable, as it mostly consists fatty tissue.

Involution of the thymus has been linked to loss of immune function in the elderly, susceptibility to infection and to cancer.

The type of malfunction falls into one or more of the following major groups:

1. hypersensitivity or allergy;
2. auto-immune disease or immunodeficiency.

Thymus medulla which secretes thymus hormones is found atrophied in Breast Cancer; while thymus cortex which produces lymphocytes is found hypertrophied in patients with Breast Cancer which suggests a define connection of this gland with oncogenesis, but it is yet to understand with clarity.[58]

Homeopathic Indications

1. Arthritis deformans; metabolic osteoarthritis.
2. Exophthalmic goitre.
3. From the earliest period of childhood to about the second year, it is at its greatest maturity. Then it gradually declines to the period of puberty, when the gonads become active.
4. If there is disturbance of the thyroid, pituitary, hypoplastic ovaries or castration after puberty, this glands hypertrophies.
5. Symptoms similar to Phosphorus.

Chapter 9

Radioactive Substances

Radiation Exposure is indeed linked with Carcinogenesis including Breast Cancer.

This was proved in a study on the victims of Hiroshima-Nagasaki Tragedy, Chernobyl Nuclear Power Plant Accident, Radium factory workers and other occupational hazards; and those who were given Radiation as a therapy.

Generally, the action is not immediate, and it takes years to develop cancer after the exposure to radioactivity.

An individual susceptibility plays an important role in development of disease.

According to the concept of drug proving, if radiation can produce Cancer, it can also cure it.

Giving radioactive substance in potentized form like Nosode as an intercurrent during the treatment of cancer is a widely accepted clinical approach.

Few of the radioactive medicines are well known while others' action is yet to be explored.

The known Radioactive Human Breast Carcinogens are:

1. X- Ray
2. Gamma Rays

3. Radium salts
4. Radioactive Iodine
5. Thorium
6. Plutonium
7. Neptunium 237
8. Radon
9. Cesium, especially Cesium Chloride

1. Radium

Radium was discovered by Marie Sklodowska Curie, a Polish chemist, and Pierre Curie, a French chemist, in 1898. Marie Curie obtained Radium from pitchblende, a material that contains Uranium.

It is an alkaline earth metal, next to Barium and analogous to it in many chemical properties. It is a radioactive element, having Thorium as a parent and Radon as a daughter. It decays into Radon emitting alpha, beta and gamma particles.

Radium had been used to make self-luminous paints for watches, aircraft instruments, military equipments, dials and other instrumentation, but has largely been replaced by Cobalt-60, a less dangerous radioactive source. A mixture of Radium and Beryllium *emits* neutrons, thus *used as a neutron source. Radium is used to produce* radon, a radioactive gas used to treat various types of Cancer.

Since Radium ulcerates skin it comes into contact with, this property has led to its use as an agent to destroy tumor.

Radium is now replaced in industrial use by safer radioactive substances after its toxicity was known by after health hazards in Radium Girls who ingested Radium while painting dials. Such ingested Radium accumulates in bones replacing its chemical analogue Calcium, starts emitting radioactive particles and harms marrow gives rise to anemia and Cancer, especially of breast, bone and blood. Being a Metaloestrogen, Radium is more likely to produce and cure Estrogen positive Breast Cancer with a tendency to metastasize to blood and bones.

Keywords: Radioactive;   Bone-Blood-Breast   Carcinogen; Metaloestrogen; Estrogen Positive Breast Cancer

Homeopathic Indications

1. A Deeper Rhus Tox.

2. < first movement; cold.

3. > by warm application.

4. Lateness in appearance of symptoms.

5. Apprehensive, depressed; fear of being alone in the dark; great desire to be with people.

6. Vivid Dreams, of fire.

7. Predominantly right - sided.

8. Intolerance of tobacco

9. Development and Regeneration Retards (Barium Symptom)

10. Weakness, vertigo, tendency to cutaneous epithelioma.

11. The pains are severe, sharp and darting in character, there may be cracking about the joints.

12. The parts may have a sensation as if they are hard and brittle and would break if moved.

13. Craves cool open air (Puls).

14. Craves pork.

15. Averse to sweets, ice cream.

16. Dryness of mouth. Metallic taste. Prickling sensation in the end of tongue.

17. Entire body feels as if a fire with sharpest kind of needle-pricks or electric shocks all over the body, with itching.

18. Sudden, lightning-like, shocking pains.

19. Electric shock through the body during sleep.
20. Effect of X-ray burns.
21. Ulcers due to Radium burns, take a long time to heal.
22. Eczematous eruptions, cracks, scaly excrescences, and wart-like outcropping, Corns, Nevus.
23. Exposure to rays causes dermatitis, proceeding to ulceration, necrosis and epithelioma.
24. As if skull too small, as if foreign body (lash) in eye, as if something dropped into trachea. Knees feel as if the bones would protrude.
25. Sciatica, neuritis, gout.
26. Nephritis, with rheumatism.
27. It has a decided action on the blood, increasing the red blood cells and reducing the white blood count.
28. Like Uranium nitrate, this remedy relieves glycosuria, and modifies diabetes mellitus. The urine is extremely acid.
29. Pruritus vulvae. Delayed and irregular menstruation and backache.
30. Leucorrhea, white and scanty, curdy and cheesy.
31. Menses last one day; then bloody leucorrhea.
32. Uterine hemorrhage, when Ipecac fails.
33. Right breast sore, relieved by hard rubbing.
34. Aggravation: Getting up. Motion. Shaving. Washing. Summer heat. Stretching parts.
35. Amelioration: Open air. Hot bath. Eating. Lying down. Cold drinks. Continued Motion (Rhus Tox). Exertion. Pressure.
36. Worse: Motion. Shaving. Washing. Smoking. Getting up.
37. Better: Open air. Hot bath. Cold drinks. Continued motion. After sleep. Pressure. Eating.
38. Relationship: Radium brom. is antidoted by Rhus venenata and Tellurium. It is followed well by Rhus ven., Sepia and Calcarea.

39. Compare to Calcarea in aggravation by wetting; and with Carbo anim. in aggravation by shaving.

2. X Ray

X Ray is a known human carcinogen according to American Cancer Society and its exposure is strongly associated with early onset of Breast Cancer.

It is a double-edged sword which is equally employed in the treatment of Breast Cancer and many other Cancers as a Radiotherapy owing to its property to "BURN".

It is delivered to the localized malignant growth (target) in order to destroy them by burning in radiotherapy.

Women with BRCA genetic mutations showed more chances to develop Breast Cancer when exposed to X ray.[59]

Keywords: Burn; Carcinogen; Early Onset Breast cancer; BRCA Mutations

Homeopathic Indications

Adynamic conditions, anemia, change in the generalcondition, for all skin and digestive complaints in a cancerous type.

History of repeated X-Ray exposure.

It counteracts the side effects of Radiation.

Suppressed symptoms after radiotherapy.

Sits in the corner alone; not wanting to do anything.

1. Mental condition upset during profuse menstruation, desires to kill somebody.
2. Suicidal disposition: throwing himself from a height.
3. General debility.
4. Emaciation.

5. Hypochromic anemia.

6. Leucocytes decreased.

7. Platelets decreased.

8. Hemorrhagic syndromes.

9. Purpura.

10. Warts, benign skin tumors.

11. Chronic itching eruptions.

12. Radiodermatitis.

13. Ingrowing nails.

14. Appetite only for cake and sweet pudding.

15. Aversion to Meat.

16. No hunger goes till he feels faint.

17. Very thirsty, thirst for cold drinks.

18. Grey teeth.

19. Heart sounds keep one awake while lying on the left side.

20. Cannot bear slightest touch, though hard pressure relieves for an instant; neuralgic pains.

21. Aggravation from the cold, from movement.

22. Amelioration from hot application.

23. Atrophy and Degeneration of Organs.

24. Thickening of Skin.

25. Rough and Scaly palms.

26. Psoriasis and itchy eczema.

27. Clumsy hands.

28. Menses dark green one day.

29. Nerve pains after mastectomy.

Chapter 10

Synthetic Remedies

Synthetic remedies are the remedies made from synthetic chemicals or products, and not from natural sources. Synthetic remedies include:

1. Cisplatin
2. Carboplatin
3. Oxaliplatin
4. Tamoxiphene
5. Flourouracil

The entire modern medicine is based upon such factory-made chemicals which are, most of the times, synthetic versions of natural active alkaloids/constituents of plant or other natural medicines.

These remedies are superior in action than natural, crude versions as they are in in their most refined, most active extract form, which can directly target the biochemical reaction with utmost precision producing fastest results.

Though they are excellent for emergency and palliation, synthetic remedies have failed to restore sick to health permanently and their prolonged use has resulted in many untoward side effects specific to particular chemicals.

They are being used in homeopathy in their potentized form to cure the side effects they have produced.

They can be also given for altered biochemical chain of reactions they are capable to produce, for deeper organic diseases, which does not yield solely to the indicated dynamic natural remedy, as a complementary medicine.

It is Dr Sarkar's novel approach to apply chemotherapeutic drugs in potentized form for fairly advanced cancer cases with paucity of symptoms or poor reaction.

Most of the drugs employed in chemotherapy produces Secondary Cancer as their side effects.

The secret is to harness their cancer-causing potential as a cancer curing principle with the exact precision, they are capable to produce, as a Complementary/Intercurrent Remedy, especially in fairly advanced cancer cases.

The side effects they produce are used as their indications on the basis of symptom similarity along with clinical findings from doctors' experience.

This is a novel concept, but clinical results, though are encouraging, demands vigorous research as Cancers has become very much common nowadays due to human exposure to synthetic chemicals and unnatural living habits.

 Relapsed, metastatic cancers due to the chemotherapy may also be considered, in first instance, as their secondary side effect.

These Cancers likely yield remedies made from artificial sources than the natural ones as their origin is unnatural.

Chemotherapeutic drugs useful for breast cancer with their side effects as indications and Dr Sarkar's observations are described below.

Platinum Based Drugs

Platinum based drugs are employed as an adjuvant or non-adjuvant chemotherapy for highly aggressive, metastatic kind of Triple Negative Breast Cancers.

They are found more effective in patients with BRCA gene mutations.

Their mode of action have been linked to its ability to crosslink with the purine bases on the DNA; interfering with DNA repair mechanisms, causing DNA damage, and subsequently inducing apoptosis in cancer cells.

They are effective for shorter duration only and have hazardous side effects.

1. Cisplatin

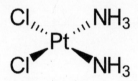

Side effects

1. Hair Loss.
2. Nausea and vomiting.
3. Myelosuppression.
4. Peripheral Neuropathy.
5. Nephrotoxicity
6. Ototoxicity, Tinnitus and Hearing loss.
7. Liver Damage.
8. Low blood counts of Ca, K, P.
9. Loss of appetite, Metallic taste in mouth.

Homeopathic Indications

1. Unable to control himself.
2. Obnoxious.
3. Dreadful dreams of suicide and accidents.
4. Desire for milk, alcohol, tobacco.
5. Blueness of hands.
6. Persistent vomiting and nausea at the terminal stage of cancer.

2. Carboplatin

Side effects

1. Constipation.
2. Mouth sores.
3. Immunosuppression.
4. Peripheral neuropathy.
5. Central neurotoxicity.
6. Ototoxicity: Symptoms include dizziness, confusion, visual changes, ringing in the ears, loss of high pitched sounds.
7. Nephrotoxicity.
8. Abnormal blood electrolyte levels (sodium, potassium, calcium).
9. Abnormal blood liver enzymes (SGOT, Alkaline phosphatase).
10. Cardiovascular events. Infrequent, heart failure, blood clots and strokes have been reported with Carboplatin use.
11. Allergic reaction.

3. Oxaliplatin

Side effects

1. Anaphylaxis and Allergic reactions.
2. Neuropathy.
3. Severe Neutropenia.
4. Pulmonary Fibrosis and Toxicities.
5. Hepatotoxicity.
6. Cardiovascular Toxicities.
7. Rhabdomyolysis.

Antiestrogen Medicines

4. Tamoxifen

Tamoxifen is a selective estrogen-receptor modulator of non-steroidal origin of triphenylethylene group of compounds.

Tamoxifen has predominantly antiestrogenic effects in the breasts while estrogenic effects in the uterus and liver.

Tamoxifen is used for the treatment of both early and advanced Estrogen receptor-positive (ER-positive or ER+) Breast Cancer in pre- and post-menopausal women.

The use of Tamoxifen is normally recommended for 10 years.

It works by disinhibiting the hypothalamic–pituitary–gonadal axis (HPG axis) via ER antagonism, thereby increasing the secretion of luteinizing hormone (LH) and follicle-stimulating hormone (FSH).

It reduces IGF 1 levels giving rise to Metabolic syndrome causing Hypertension, Hyperlipidemia, Diabetes and Obesity.

It also inhibits Protein Kinase C impairing memory and learning causing mental disorders.

Side Effects

1. Lower limb lymphedema.
2. Embolism, blood clots and deep vein thrombosis (DVT).
3. Osteoporosis.
4. Rapid increase in triglyceride concentration in the blood.
5. Memory Impairment.
6. Obesity.

It is a known carcinogen which can produce Uterine Cancer and Contralateral Breast Cancer.

Homeopathic Indications

1. Increased Hunger.
2. Complementary to Hydrastis.
3. Metastasis to Liver, Hepatocellular Cancer and very fatty liver with decreased visual activities with hot flushes.
4. Atrophy of Vagina.
5. Hair loss.
6. Nausea and Vomiting.
7. DVT, Pituitary embolism with prolonged us of OCP.
8. Memory impairment.
9. Endometrial Cancer; Premature Ovarian Failure.
10. After radiation-operation recurrence of lump in another breast.
11. Prolonged use of OCP's.

5. Fluorouracil

Fluorouracil or 5-FU (trademark Efudex) is a drug, i.e. a Pyrimidine analogue, used in the treatment of Cancer.

It is a thymine inhibitor necessary for DNA replication and works through irreversible inhibition of Thymidylate synthase.

It belongs to the family of drug called Antimetabolites.

Homeopathic Indications

1. Lycopodium like constitution + Cancer of Breast.
2. Used mainly as an intercurrent remedy.
3. Complementary to Lycopodium.
4. < Evening.
5. >Warm drinks.
6. <By Cold.
7. Concomitant dry thick skin and loose stools.
8. Myelosuppression.
9. Mucositis.
10. Dermatitis.
11. Diarrhea.
12. Premalignant Breast condition.
13. Inflammatory Breast Cancer.
14. Acute Cerebellar Syndrome; Ataxia, Nystagmus and Dysmetria.

Chapter 11

New Plant Remedies For Cancer

1. Agrimony Eupatorium

Agrimony is a wellknown Chinese remedy for Liver problems, Diabetes and Cancer. Ali et. al 2013 have demonstrated its cytotoxic properties in-vitro.[60] It contains 11 antineoplastic constituents. It proves to be effective for bone cancer, namely sarcoma 180 and Ehrlich ascites carcinoma. It promotes the Growth of Healthy Cells.

Homeopathic Indications

1. It has masked troubles; is anxious and worried internally, has forced cheerfulness externally.

2. Hides one's sufferings, even though suffering internal torment; is full of interest in life; is a daredevil and reckless in all the ways.

3. It is active and restless, always on the move, requires little sleep.

4. Makes one believe he is happy and cheerful, while at heart one prefers death, seeks excitement, desires, stimulants and is worried by an imaginary prosecutor.

5. Suppression, over-compliance and denial of emotions.

6. Desire to not let others down and burden them with their personal problems. Intend to spread cheer and uplift others. Tendency not to express strong emotions which could bring disharmony or strife to oneself or others.

7. Grief or other forms of disappointment. Resentment or guilt which are not being worked through. Unresolved conflicts or trauma. Inner restlessness, a sense of boredom. Often finds some relief in drugs, entertainment, or other forms of diversion, and is interested in the occult and magic.

8. Distress due to quarrels and bring unhappiness.

9. In any condition where the patient holds the breath to stop the pain, this causes the release of endo-morphine, the body's own opiates which suppresses the pain.

10. Hepatitis and cirrhosis of liver from chronic alcoholism, fat metabolism (cirrhosis starts from lower lobe of liver) tension and suppressed anger are associated with liver and gall bladder.

11. Incontinence following passing of stone.

12. Pain in the region of kidneys from any cause, pain specially in the right side of kidney.

13. Altitude sickness.

14. Constipation.

15. Relieves Pain of Cancer.

16. Abdominal distention, regurgitation, dysphasia.

17. Pulmonary abscess.

18. Hematemesis.

19. Hemorrhoids.

20. Painful kidney region.

21. Cough leading to spurting of urine.

2. Allium Sativa

Garlic, another herb widely used in culinary, from Liliaceae family (Ornithogalum Umbellata, Sarsaparilla), is well-known for its anticancer properties as it is found to prevent rate of cancer in people who used to consume it daily in food.

Allicin, Sulphur compounds and Selenium present in garlic are excellent anticancer compounds.

It is found to prevent liver from Tamoxifen toxicity.

It binds with Alfa Estrogen Receptor and found to be effective against MCF 7 Breast Cancer lines.[61]

A study on Female rats revealed that rats who were fed fresh garlic became immune to Breast Cancer, injecting millions of cancer cells into mice, and no tumor developed in the rats resulting in 100 % effectiveness.

Out of 194 patients of lip ca 184 were cured simply by rubbing fresh garlic several times a day over the wound.

Homeopathic Indications:

1. Symptoms of sympathetic excess of hyper adrenalins (anxiety, nervousness, high blood pressure, sweating, rapid heartbeat).

2. Premature ageing, memory loss.

3. Fear: medicine, of not being able to bear any kind of.

4. Fear: poisoned, of being.

5. A wonderful remedy for psoriasis.

6. Old People: Fleshy, Dyslectic.

7. High Living: Gluttony; Meat Eater.

8. Swelling, Dropsical: Fever, Intermittent, After Protracted, In Marshy Districts.

9. Genital: Eruption: Pustules: Menses during.

10. Empyema of maxillary sinus.

11. Menstruation: Extreme weakness she could hardly do anything, except lie still and not talk. cold sweat extreme thirst, faintness, sometimes violent and diarrhea, morning sickness.

12. Éruption in Breast, menses during.

13. Sleep prevented by thirst.

3. Althea Officinalis

Common name: Marshmallow; Family: Malvalaceae (Chocolate family).

Its mucilaginous root has been used since centuries as a nutritive and culinary delicacy.

It is an old herb used in Islamic-Arabian Medicine for Cancer and wound healing.

The root is full of antioxidants, the root contains substance potent to fight against plant fungi and pathogens, it contains coumarins which are known for their anticancer potential and antiestrogenic activities.

Homeopathic Indications

1. Best friend during chemotherapy.

2. Inflexible, narrow-minded, emotionally rigid or unfeeling, hard-hearted, insensitive, unsympathetic.

3. Lips red; tongue red, glazed, burnished, horizontal, Cracks with coating.

4. Swollen, hard, indurated glands.

5. Prevents formation of pus.

6. Dry cough, constipation, systemic dryness.

7. Arthritis, High BP; Hematuria, Hemorrhoids.

Particular Indications

Mind (including Senses, Nerves, Emotions, Personality)

1. Inflexible, narrow-minded, emotionally rigid or unfeeling.
2. Hardhearted, insensitive, unsympathetic.

Head

1. Eyes, sore, inflamed (external).

Mucous membrane

1. Lips red, dry, sometimes with a slight white powder around them.
2. Tongue red, dry, glazed, burnished, horizontal cracks; with dry coating.
3. Irritated, inflamed, hot, dry mucosa.
4. Sore throat.

Lymphatic system

1. Swollen, hard, indurated glands.

Respiratory system

1. Dry cough in the throat or upper bronchus; in children; worse at night.
2. Bronchitis and asthma.
3. Whooping cough.
4. Emphysema.

Digestive system

1. Soothing and anti-inflammatory to the digestive tract; acid stomach, burning (capsules).
2. Over-acidity, ulcers, gastric, duodenal, mucus colitis (roots).
3. Low enzyme production (leaves) with gastric acidity
4. Diarrhea, dysentery, Crohn's disease colitis

5. Constipation.

6. Hemorrhoids (external).

Excretory system

1. Painful, scanty urination; soothes the passage of stones.

2. Cystitis, strangury, hematuria.

3. Gravel.

Female reproductive system

1. Lactation: nipples, sore (external).

Musculoskeletal

1. Arthritis in knees; with dry mucosa, tongue red, dry, latitudinal cracks (cured).

Skin

1. Sores, ulcers, burns, boils, and inflamed skin (external).

2. Skin red, dry, with white powder exfoliating.

Others

1. High blood pressure with water retention.

2. Diabetes.

3. Side effects of Chemotherapy.

4. Thirst with copious urination or no thirst with systemic dryness.

4. Andrographis Paniculata

It is a well-known Ayurvedic Medicine from Plant Order, Lamiales; also known as Kalmegh in Sanskrit.

Andrographis is a bitter tasting herb.

According to Memorial Sloan Kettering Cancer Institute and findings of multiple research studies, it strongly acts as an anti-cancer/anti-metastatic agent.

It corrects COX 2 and several Interleukin pathways and also found to be effective against Liver, Multiple Myeloma, Gastric and Breast Cancer as well as HIV.

It is effective for prevention and treatment of Cancer, and also to counter chemotherapy toxicity in humans.

In a study in 1999, Roswell Park Institute, New York confirmed its anticancer activity as well.

It is proved to be more potent than Paclitaxel in Breast Cancer and Multi-drug resistant tumor.

It also promotes phagocytosis, preventing further metastasis.

It is indicated for trophoblastic tumor as well.

Homeopathic Indications

(Ref: 'the Drugs of Hindustan' by Dr Ghosh)

1. It is a liver remedy.
2. Mental depression and despondency.
3. Bad taste in the mouth.
4. Bitter and putrid taste over the tongue.
5. Constipation.
6. Scantiness of stools.
7. Burning sensation and heat in eyes, face hands and feet, especially in the palms.
8. Sometimes, the patient likes cold application and sometimes, he dislikes them.
9. Changeableness of symptoms.
10. During fever, there is intermingling of chilliness and burning sensation.
11. Heaviness of the whole body for which the patient walks slowly or does not like to move.

5. Asparagus Racemosus

Asparagus, a plant of Liliaceae family, a well-known Ayurvedic Herb called "Shatavari" in Sanskrit.

"Shatavari" may be translated as "100 spouses", implying its ability to increase fertility and vitality in females.

In Ayurveda, this amazing herb is known as the "Queen of herbs", because it promotes love and devotion.

Shatavari is the main Ayurvedic rejuvenative tonic for females.

It is known for its ulcer healing potential.

It prevents threatened abortion and restores menstrual health is a potent galactagogue.

It contains phytoestrogen which is being proved efficacious in a research study on Estrogen positive Breast Cancer targeting Estrogen Receptors.[62]

It is found to inhibit Sarcoma 180, Leukemia, Lung and Breast Carcinoma.

6. Astragalus

Astragalus is another remedy with estrogenic action from Pea family (DDx Trifolium Pratensis).

It is a well-known Chinese Medicine used since 2000 years for its tonic effects and various health benefits.

It is seen is very promising herbal drug for Cancer.

According to Memorial Sloan Kettering Cancer Institute, it is found to reduce need and side effects of Chemotherapy; to prolong progression free survival time in Cancer patients; remove Cancer related fatigue. It is also found efficacious against various Cancers including Breast Cancer in various research studies.[63]

It also stimulates production of interferon.

More or less specific, it helps to counteract the immune damaging effect of chemotherapy.

The alkaloid 'swainsonine' inhibits metastasis of melanoma.

Howard University Cancer Center performed a study on mice with lung carcinoma by adding swainsonine in their drinking water. It was observed that within 24 hours, it inhibited 80% of tumor colonies.

It stimulates spleen cells to exercise anti-metastatic effect.

It is also effective in stimulating hemopoietic factors and interleukin production.

It potentiates the activity of chemotherapeutic agents, inhibits recurrence of malignancies, prolongs survival, reduces adverse toxicities of radiotherapy and anti-neoplastic agent (Mitomycin, Cisplatin, Cyclophosphamide and 5-Flurouracil).

Diarrhea, fatigue, spontaneous sweating, lack of appetite, frequent cold, shortness of breath, wasting disorder, chronic ulceration and sore, numbness and paralysis of limbs, edema.

7. Celastrus Candense:

Celastrus is one of the ten herbs of Dr Ely G. Jones' Cancer Syrup.

Its invasive Asian variant, Celastrus Orbiculatus, is a well-known Chinese medicine uses since years for the treatment of Cancer.

It is an anti-angiogenic medicine and works over Vascular Endothelial Growth Factor (VGEF) and have produced apoptosis in Hepatocarcinoma in-vivo and vitro.[67]

In Ayurveda, it is called 'Jyotishmati' and used as a nervine tonic and neurological disorders.

Celastrus S. is also found producing apoptosis and autophagy in Breast Cancer cells.[68]

It acts on small intestines in order to improve absorption and nutrition.

It is not only indicated in wasting and withering, but also in congestion, edema due to weakness of lymphatic system surrounding intestine and kidney.

It is useful in swollen, indurated glands, cracked breasts, mastitis, and Breast Cancer.

It is good for Dry Skin.

It also acts on Hypothalamus.

8. Citrus Aurantia

Sour Orange is a known traditional Chinese medicine for various types of Cancer.

It is found antiestrogenic, binds to the Estradiol Receptors causing breast cancer and suggested as a useful medicine for Estrogen Positive Breast Cancer and Osteoporosis in a study at Malta.[69]

It enhances cytotoxic ability of T–cells and natural killer cells in their ability to prevent metastasis.

It neutralizes the effects of Tamoxifen as well as used to relieve Cancer pain.

9. Curcuma Longa

The active alkaloid, Curcumin, is one of the most potent anti-cancer phytochemicals and is widely used as a natural supplement in treatment of Cancer globally.

Homoeopathic Indications

1. H/o INJURY.
2. Stammering.
3. It causes gall bladder to contract and secrete.
4. Inhibits fungi.
5. ER + BREAST CANCER.
6. INHIBITORY EFFECT ON GROWTH OF HUMAN BREAST CANCER MCF7 CELLS INDUCED BY ESTROGENIC PESTICIDES.
7. Stomach Cancer.
8. Liver cancer (Glutathione-s-transferase activity increases).

Curcuma Aromatica

For regression of precancerous lesion of palate due to smoking.

10. Inula

This is a medicine from Compositae family (Arnica, Bellis Per).

Like other family members of the same plant, it is also found very useful against various Cancers including Breast and Pancreas.

There have been many studies which confirmed its anticancer role including a Chinese one which confirmed its role against Triple Negative Kind of Breast Cancer.[64]

History of Injury is one of the confirming points.

1. Lungs and Breast Cancer.
2. Cough, with abundant thick expectoration, with weakness of digestive tract.
3. Dry cough at night, aggravated by lying down, with difficult breathing.
4. General languor, debility.

5. Chronic skin affections.

6. Engorged glands.

7. Leucorrhea.

8. Allied in chemical constitution to Kreosote.

9. Something alive moving about internally,

10. Another peculiar sensation is as though someone was poking him with a finger in various parts of the body.

11. Painful, he awake with clenched teeth.

12. Numerous sticking pains as with pins or a knife.

11. Juglans Nigra

Common name: Black walnut.

Juglans Nigra constitutes antioxidants, and in potent, cytotoxic medicine owing to its capacity to alter Reactive Oxidation Stress.

Black and green walnut both contains an active constituent, Juglone, which is well established as an anti-cancer phytochemical.

It is a PIN 1 inhibitor.[65]

PIN 1 is a proto-oncogene which regulates several proteins involved in cancer initiation and progression[66] and its inhibition has resulted in tumor disappearance.

Pin 1 inhibition is much desired target of cancer researchers and Juglone holds one such promise.

Juglans is found effective against many kinds of cancers like liver, colorectal and Breast.

It is found useful for Autointoxication—toxins uptake from constipated bowels; leaky bowel syndrome—or dysbiosis. It treats opposite conditions—malabsorption, helps assimilation of nutrients, reduces unhealthy fatty acids from blood stream. It is also indicated in Goiter, hypothyroidism, caused by low cellular metabolism, or due to faulty liver. Iodine is concentrated and secreted by the breasts and are essential for breast health. deficiency may lead to fibrocystic breast and breast cancer.

Homoeopathic Indications

Too much under the influence of another person, thought.

12. Lilium Longiflorum

Lilium longiflorum is a species with beautiful, large, white flowers which grows in Asia Minor and the Mediterranean area.

It is a bulbous plant with beautifully scented flowers used in the floral industry and folk medicine.

The plant contains a number of bioactive substances that exhibit anti-inflammatory, cytotoxic, hepatoprotective and antitumor effects.

A study at Babylon University has stated that Lilium alkaloids extract can be used as an efficient traditional anticancer alternative medicine, at moderately low dosage.[70]

It is from a Liliaceae family; the other famous anti-cancer medicines from the same family include Ornithogalum, Sarsaparilla and Allium Sativum.

Homeopathic Indications

1. Breast Cancer, metastasized to lungs.
2. Easter Lily is an important remedy to help those individuals who feel a great inner tension between their sexuality and spirituality.

13. Lonicera Japonica

Common name: Honeysuckle

Homeopathic Indications

1. Inhibits Sarcoma 180.
2. Leukemia.
3. Lung and Breast Cancer.

14. Nigella Sativa

Nigella is one the most revered medicinal seeds in history.

The best seeds come from Egypt where they grow under almost perfect conditions in oasis and are watered until the seed pods form.

Black cumin seeds were found in the tomb of Tutankhamun.

Though black cumin seeds are mentioned in the Bible as well as in the words of the Prophet Mohammed, they were not carefully researched until about forty years ago.

Since then, more than 200 studies have been conducted in universities.

The first major study of Nigella sativa in prevention and treatment of Cancer was performed by scientists at Cancer Immuno-Biology Laboratory of Hilton Head Island, South Carolina.

1. **Colon Cancer**: In cell studies, black seed has been found to have anti-cancer properties, inhibiting the growth of colon cancer cells specifically.
2. **Breast Cancer** - A few studies have linked a thymoquinone extract from Nigella Sativa to reduce Breast tumor growth and increased apoptosis (cell death) in Breast Cancer cells.
3. **Brain Cancer** - A study published in the online journa,l 'PLoS One' indicates thymoquinone from black seed can induce cell death in glioblastoma cells. Glioblastoma is one of the most aggressive Brain Tumors of all.

4. **Oral Cancer** – Research indicates thymoquinone from Nigella Sativa is able to induce cell apoptosis in oral cancer cells.

5. **Radiation Damage Control** – The active compound, thymoquinone, has been found to protect brain tissue from radiation-induced damage.

6. **Parkinson's Disease** – An extract of thymoquinone from black seed, was shown to protect neurons from toxicity associated with Parkinson's disease and dementia in a study published in *Neuroscience Letters*.

7. **Cervical Cancer** – In a cervical cancer cell line, extracts of thymoquinone were able to trigger apoptosis or cell death, slow Cancer progression, and stop the spread of the Cancer.

8. **Pancreatic cancer** – Thymoquinone +Gemcitabine + Oxaliplatin induced 60-80 % apoptosis while only Gemcitabine +Oxaliplatin induced 16-20 % apoptosis in cell lines in a study.

15. Trapa Bicurnus

Common name: Water Chestnut, Paniphal.

Chinese name – LING SHUI.

Homeopathic Indications

1. Breast Cancer; Stomach Cancer; Esophagus Cancer; Cervical Cancer.

2. Gastric ulcer.

3. Infantile head sore.

16. Trichosanthes/Dhundhul

Homeopathic Indications

1. Chinese research has proven the anticancer effects.

2. Nasopharyngeal Cancer.

3. Cough with blood steaked sputum.

4. It regulates over utilization of estrogen and testosterone.

5. Estrogen+ Breast Cancer, uterine and prostate Cancer.

Glossary

5-Flurouracil- (5FU)- A pyrimidine analogue used as an antineoplastic agent to treat multiple solid tumors.

Adrenal crisis- A potentially life-threatening medical condition requiring immediate emergency treatment.

Aflatoxin- Poisonous carcinogens that are produced by certain molds which grow in soil, decaying vegetation, hay, and grains.

Agaricocyte- A class of fungi in the division Basidiomycota.

Allicin- A compound produced when garlic is crushed or chopped. It is available in dietary supplement form, it's been found to reduce inflammation and offer antioxidant benefits.

Alpha Estrogen Receptors- (ERα), also known as NR3A1 (nuclear receptor subfamily 3, group A, member 1), is one of two main types of estrogen receptor, a nuclear receptor that is activated by the sex hormone estrogen

Andropogen- Alternative name of anantherum muriaticum.

Aniline- An organic compound with the formula C_6H_5NH, its main use is the manufacture of precursors to polyurethane and other industrial chemicals.

Anthraquinone- A polycyclic aromatic hydrocarbon derived from anthracene or phthalic anhydride which isused in the manufacture of dyes, in the textile and pulp industries, and as a bird repellant.

Aphrodisiac- A substance that increases sexual desire, sexual pleasure, and/or sexual behavior.

APL- Acute promyelocytic leukemia (APML, APL) is a subtype of acute myeloid leukemia (AML), a cancer of the white blood cells.

Arachidonic Acid - An unsaturated fatty acid found ubiquitously in plasma membranes, where it is bound to phospholipid. Its metabolism produces prostaglandins, prostacyclins, thromboxanes, and leukotrienes.

Aristolochic acid- A carcinogenic, mutagenic, and nephrotoxic phytochemical, commonly found in the flowering plant family, Aristolochiaceae (birthworts).

Aromatase Enzyme- Also called estrogen synthetase or estrogen synthase, is an enzyme responsible for a key step in the biosynthesis of estrogens. It is CYP19A1, a member of the cytochrome P450 superfamily, which are monooxygenases that catalyze many reactions involved in steroidogenesis.

Aromatic compounds- Also known as arenas or aromatics, they are chemical compounds that contain conjugated planar ring systems with delocalized pi-electron clouds, instead of discrete alternating single and double bonds.

Arsenicosis- Arsenic poisoning.

Benzyl quinoline alkaloids- Found within the structures of a wide variety of plant natural products, collectively referred to as benzylisoquinoline alkaloids.

Berberine- A quaternary ammonium salt from the protoberberine group of benzylisoquinoline alkaloids found in such plants as Berberis.

Beta Estrogen Receptors- (ER-β), also known as NR3A2 (nuclear receptor subfamily 3, group A, member 2), is one of two main types of estrogen receptor, a nuclear receptor which is activated by the sex hormone estrogen

Boletus- Boletus is a genus of mushroom-producing fungi, comprising over 100 species.

BRCA gene- The BRCA genes are tumour suppressor genes which produce proteins that help repair damaged DNA, keeping the genetic material of the cell stable.

Bufotanins-(5-HO-DMT, bufotenine) is a tryptamine derivative related to the neurotransmitter serotonin. It is an alkaloid found in the skin of some species of toads, mushrooms, higher plants, and mammals.

Camouflage- The use of any combination of materials, coloration, or illumination for concealment, either by making animals or objects hard to see, or by disguising them as something else

Cannabinoid receptors- Located throughout the body, these receptors are part of the endocannabinoid system, involved in a variety of physiological processes including appetite, pain-sensation, mood, and memory.

Carboplatin- A chemotherapeutic drug which is a heavy metal compound that inhibits synthesis of RNA, DNA, and protein in cells.

CD4-CD8-CD12-CD19- Clusters of differentiation - T cell and B cell markers

Chimaphilin- An active compound separated from pyrola, possesses the highly efficient antitumor activities.

Circadian rhythm- Biological clock, roughly 24-hour cycle in the physiological processes of living beings, including plants, animals, fungi and cyanobacteria.

Cisplatin- Cisplatin, cisplatinum or cis-diamminedichloroplatinum(II) (CDDP) is a platinum-based chemotherapy drug used to treat various types of cancers, including sarcomas.

Citric acid cycle- The citric acid cycle – also known as the TCA or the Krebs cycle – is a series of chemical reactions used by all aerobic organisms to release stored energy through the oxidation ofacetyl-CoA derived from carbohydrates, fats, and proteins, into adenosine triphosphate and carbon dioxide.

Conduritol- 1,2,3,4-cyclohexenetetrol is any of the organic compounds with chemical formula $C_6H_{10}O_4$, that can be seen as derivatives of cyclohexene with four hydroxyl groups (OH).

Coniine- It is a piperidine alkaloid, (based on the piperidine structure). Its effects are similar to that of Nicotine (a pyrrolidine alkaloid)

Convallotoxin- It is a digitalis-like compound (DLC), which is mainly used as a cardiac glycoside since it can inhibit the Na^+,K^+-ATPase in congestive heart failure or arrythmias, which causes an inotropic effect, same as many other digitalis like compounds.

Coumarin- It is a compound of cinnamon that has been reported to possess pharmacological activity, such as, anti-inflammatory, antioxidant, antihyperglycemic, antiadipogenic, antibacterial, and anticancer properties.

COX 2 pathway- The cyclooxygenase (COX) enzyme system is the major **pathway** catalyzing the conversion of arachidonic acid into prostaglandins (PGs) here COX-2 is an inducible enzyme as it is produced under certain specific conditions like inflammation.

Curcumin- It is a bright yellow chemical produced by Curcuma longa plants. It is the principal curcuminoid of turmeric (Curcuma longa), a member of the ginger family, Zingiberaceae.

Cyclophosphamide- It is a cancer medication that interferes with the growth and spread of cancer cells in the body and suppresses the immune system.

Cytochrome C Oxidase- (COX) is a terminal oxidase, composed of four catalytic subunits that functions to transport electrons from reduced cytochrome c to the final electron acceptor oxygen molecule.

Cytostatic- It is the inhibition of cell growth and multiplication.

Dexamethasone- is a steroid that prevents the release of substances in the body that cause inflammation.

Diterpenoid alkaloids – These are an unusual group of "secondary metabolites" produced by plants; they can be derived biogenetically from an isoprenoid pathway which in the early stages is probably similar to that used in gibberellic acid biosynthesis.

Doxorubicin- It is a type of chemotherapy drug called an anthracycline. It slows or stops the growth of cancer cells by blocking an enzyme called topo-isomerase 2. Cancer cells need this enzyme to divide and grow.

Ehrlich ascites- Ehrlich ascites carcinoma is a spontaneous murine mammary adenocarcinoma adapted to ascites form and carried in outbred mice by serial intraperitoneal (i/p) passages

Endomorphins-   They are considered to be natural opioid neurotransmitters central to pain relief.

Endophytes- These are organisms, often fungi and bacteria, that live between living plant cells. The relationship that they establish with the plant varies from symbiotic to bordering on pathogenic.

Epigenetic- It is the study of heritable phenotype changes that do not involve alterations in the DNA sequence.

ER- negative- It describes cells that do not have a protein to which the hormone estrogen will bind. Cancer cells that are estrogen receptor negative do not need estrogen to grow, and usually do not stop growing when treated with hormones that block estrogen from binding.

ER- Positive- This means the cancer cells grow in response to the hormone estrogen.

ERK-MAPK pathway- It is a chain of proteins in the cell that communicates a signal from a receptor on the surface of the cell to the DNA in the nucleus of the cell.

Estradiol- (E2), also spelled estradiol, is an estrogen steroid hormone.

Estriole- (E3), also spelled ostiole, is a steroid, a weak estrogen.

Estrone- (E1), also spelled oestrone, is a steroid, a weak estrogen

FER- Fer protein is a member of the FPS/FES family of nontrans membrane receptor tyrosine kinases. It regulates cell-cell adhesion and mediates signaling from the cell surface to the cytoskeleton via growth factor receptors.

Flavonoids – A group of plant metabolites thought to provide health benefits through cell signaling pathways and antioxidant effects.

Fluoxetine- A selective serotonin reuptake inhibitor (SSRI) antidepressant

Galactagogue- It is a substance that promotes lactation in humans and other animals.

Gemcitabine- It is a chemotherapy medication used to treat a number of types of cancer.

Gemmules- These are internal buds found in sponges and are involved in asexual reproduction.

Glucosides- It is derived from glucose.

Haustorium- It is a rootlike structure or a structure that grows into or around another structure to absorb water or nutrients.

HB-EGFs -Heparin Binding Epidermal Growth Factors- A member of the EGF family of proteins that in humans is encoded by the *HBEGF* gene is synthesized as a membrane-anchored mitogenic and chemotactic glycoprotein.

Herceptin positive breast cancer- HER2-positive breast cancer is a breast cancer that tests positive for a protein called human epidermal growth factor receptor 2 (HER2), which promotes the growth of cancer cells.

Huachansu- It is a traditional Chinese medicine extracted from the skin of the Bufo toad that is believed by some to slow the spread of cancerous cells.

Hydrastine-   It is an alkaloid. Hydrolysis of hydrastine yields hydrastinine, which was patented by Bayer as a haemostatic drug.

IGF1 AND IGF 2- (IGFs) are proteins with high sequence similarity to insulin. It consists of two cell-surface receptors (IGF1R and IGF2R), two ligands (Insulin-like growth factor 1 (IGF-1) and Insulin-like growth factor 2 (IGF-2)), a family of seven high-affinity IGF-binding proteins .

IL 8 pathways- Interleukin-8 (IL-8), alternatively known as CXCL8, is a proinflammatory CXC chemokine.

Indirubins- A chemical compound most often produced as a byproduct of bacterial metabolism.

Interleukins- (IL) are a type of cytokine. They play essential roles in the activation and differentiation of immune cells, as well as proliferation, maturation, migration, and adhesion.

Kaempferols- A natural flavanol a type of flavonoid, found in a variety of plants and plant-derived foods. acts as an antioxidant by reducing oxidative stress.

Laccata- Commonly known as the deceiver, or waxy laccaria, is a white-spore species of small edible mushroom

Leukoplakia- A condition that involves white patches or spots on the inside of the mouth. It can be caused by chewing tobacco, heavy smoking, and alcohol use.

Lycoctonine- A plant alkaloid and a precursor to the ABC ring system of taxoids.

MCF 7 Breast Cancer lines- MCF-7 is a Breast Cancer cell line isolated in 1970 from a 69-year-old Caucasian woman.[1] MCF-7 is the acronym of Michigan Cancer Foundation-7, referring to the institute in Detroit where the cell line was established in 1973 by Herbert Soule and co-workers.

MDR cancers- Multi-drug resistant cancers.

Melatonin Receptors- These are G protein-coupled receptors (GPCR) which bind melatonin. Melatonin secretion by the pineal gland has circadian rhythmicity regulated by the suprachiasmatic nucleus (SCN).

Melittin- It is the main component and the major pain producing substance of honeybee and is a basic peptide consisting of 26 amino acids.

Metaloestrogen- A class of inorganic xenoestrogens which can affect the gene expression of human cells responding to estrogen.

Methylmercury- A type of mercury, a metal that is liquid at room temperature.

Mycorrhiza- A symbiotic association between a fungus and a plant.

Mycotoxins- Toxic compounds that are naturally produced by certain types of moulds (fungi)

Nicotine Acetylcholine Receptors- nAChRs, are receptor polypeptides that respond to the neurotransmitter acetylcholine. Nicotinic receptors also respond to drugs as the agonist nicotine.

OCP- Oral contraceptive pills.

Oxaliplatin- A platinum-based chemotherapy drug in the same family as cisplatin and carboplatin.

p53 gene – The TP53 gene provides instructions for making a protein called tumor protein p53 (or p53). This protein acts as a tumor suppressor.

Paclitaxel- A chemotherapeutic medication used to treat a number of types of cancer.

Pheromones- Chemicals capable of acting like hormones outside the body of the secreting individual, to impact the behavior of the receiving individuals.

Phoenix Rising Pathway- A mechanism through which the apoptotic cell would initiate cell division in the adjacent to compensate the loss.

Phospholipase A2- t cleaves phospholipids producing lysophospholipids and free fatty acids, was originally identified as an intracellular protein involved in cell signaling and in the production of free fatty acids, such as arachidonic acid.

Phytoestrogen- (Plant estrogens) are substances that occur naturally in plants. They have a similar chemical structure to our own body's estrogen (one of the main female hormones), and are able to bind to the same receptors that our own estrogen does.

PIN 1 inhibitor- PIN1 has been shown to be a proto-oncogene whose protein product regulates several proteins involved in cancer initiation and progression and its inhibition has resulted in tumor disappearance.

Piperidine- A widely used building block and chemical reagent in the synthesis of organic compounds, including pharmaceuticals.

Piassaba- Any of a genus (Chimaphila, especially C. umbellata) of evergreen herbs of the wintergreen family (Pyrolaceae) with astringent leaves used as a tonic and diuretic.

Pitchblende- A form of the mineral uraninite occurring in brown or black masses and containing radium.

Pokeweed Mitogen- A common laboratory reagent for stimulating proliferation of B and T lymphocytes.

Polyandrous- A form of polygamy in which a woman takes two or more husbands at the same time.

Progesterone negative Breast Cancer- Describes cells that do not have a protein to which the hormone progesterone will bind. Cancer cells that are progesterone receptor negative do not need progesterone to grow, and usually do not stop growing when treated with hormones that block progesterone from binding.

Progesterone positive Breast Cancer- Describes cells that have a protein to which the hormone progesterone will bind. Cancer cells that are progesterone receptor positive need progesterone to grow and will usually stop growing when treated with hormones that block progesterone from binding.

Prostaglandin- (PG) are a group of physiologically active lipid compounds called eicosanoids having diverse hormone-like effects and are derived enzymatically from the fatty acid arachidonic acid.

Protoanemonin- (Sometimes called anemonol or ranunculol) It is a toxin found in all plants of the buttercup family.

Psychedelic- A class of drug whose primary action is to trigger psychedelic experiences via serotonin receptor agonism.

Pyridine- A colorless liquid. It is an aromatic compound similar to benzene.

Pyrrole- A colorless volatile liquid that darkens readily upon exposure to air and is usually purified by distillation immediately before use.

ROS- Chemically reactive chemical species containing oxygen. Examples include peroxides, superoxide, hydroxyl radical, singlet oxygen, and alpha oxygen.

Rubefacient- A substance for topical application that produces redness of the skin.

Rubidomycin- A new antibiotic with cytostatic properties.

Sarcoma 180 - S180- a murine Sarcoma cancer cell line. It has been commonly used in cancer research due to its rapid growth and proliferation in mice.

Sesquiterpenoid Lactone- A class of sesquiterpenoids that contain a lactone ring. They are most often found in plants of the family Asteraceae, Umbelliferae and Magnoliaciae.

Solasodine- A poisonous alkaloid chemical compound that occurs in plants of the family Solanaceae.

Steroidal cardiac glucosides- A class of organic compounds that increase the output force of the heart and increase its rate of contractions by acting on the cellular sodium-potassium ATPase pump. They are selective steroidal glycosides and are important drugs for the treatment of heart failure and cardiac rhythm disorders.

Sunitinib- A cancer medicine that interferes with the growth and spread of cancer cells in the body.

Swainsonine- An indolizidine alkaloid. It is a potent inhibitor of Golgi alpha-mannosidase II, an immunomodulator, and a potential chemotherapy drug.

Tamoxifen- The oldest and most-prescribed selective estrogen receptor modulator (SERM) it is the first hormonal therapy medicine choice for postmenopausal women.

Taxane- A class of diterpenes. They were originally identified from plants of the genus *Taxus* (yews), and feature a taxadiene core. Paclitaxel (Taxol) and docetaxel (Taxotere) are widely used as chemotherapy agents.

Teratogen - An agent or factor which causes malformation of an embryo.

Terpenes- Any of a large group of volatile unsaturated hydrocarbons found in the essential oils of plants, especially conifers and citrus trees.

Thermophiles- An organism—a type of extremophile—that thrives at relatively high temperatures, between 41 and 122 °C (106 and 252 °F).

Thymoquinone- A phytochemical compound found in the plant Nigella sativa. ... A 2016 study suggests thymoquinone may have opioid tolerance-reduction effects.

Triple Negative Breast Cancer- Cancer that tests negative for estrogen receptors, progesterone receptors, and excess HER2 protein. These results mean the growth of the cancer is not fueled by the hormones estrogen and progesterone, or by the HER2 protein.

TRPA 1 receptors- Transient receptor potential cation channel, subfamily A, member 1, also known as transient receptor potential ankyrin 1 or TRPA1, is a protein that in humans is encoded by the TRPA1 (and in other species by the Trpa1) gene. TRPA1 is an ion channel located on the plasma membrane of many human and animal cells

Vegetovascular dystonia- Features of different ailments. in the form of psychological disorders: extreme fatigue, psychological vulnerability, anxiety and fear followed by disorders of the heart, blood vessels and the peripheral nervous system.

VGEF- Vascular endothelial growth factor, originally known as vascular permeability factor, is a signal protein produced by cells that stimulates the formation of blood vessels.

Vincristine- A chemotherapeutic drug that belongs to a group of drugs called vinca alkaloids. Vincristine works by stopping the cancer cells from separating into 2 new cells.

Zearalenone- (ZEN), also known as RAL and F-2 mycotoxin, is a potent estrogenic metabolite produced by some Fusarium and Gibberella species.

Bibliography

1. Wada, K., & Yamashita, H. (2019). Cytotoxic Effects of Diterpenoid Alkaloids Against Human Cancer Cells. Molecules (Basel, Switzerland), 24(12), 2317. doi:10.3390/molecules24122317

2. Liang, Xiao-Xia & Tang, Pei & Chen, Qiao-Hong & Wang, Feng-Peng. (2012). Synthesis of Taxane ABC Tricyclic Skeleton from Lycoctonine. Natural product communications. 7. 697-703.

3. Chen, Feng & Wang, Xi & Kim, Hyun-jin. (2003). Antioxidant, Anticarcinogenic and Termiticidal Activities of Vetiver Oil.

4. Aristolochic Acid As A Probable Human Cancer Hazard In Herbal Remedies: A Review.

5. Pmid:1211062012110620; Doi 10.1093/Mutage/17.4.265

6. https://www.ncbi.nlm.nih.gov/pmc/articles/PMC6540632/ Z.Wu Et Alnaturally Occurring Sesquiterpene Lactone-Santonin, Exerts Anticancer Effects In Multi-Drug Resistant Breast Cancer Cells By Inducing Mitochondrial Mediated Apoptosis, Caspase Activation, Cell Cycle Arrest, And By Targeting Ras/Raf/Mek/Erk Signaling Pathway

7. Benarba, B., Elmallah, A., & Pandiella, A. (2019). Bryonia aqueous extract induces apoptosis and G2/M cell cycle arrest in MDA MB 231 breast cancer cells. Molecular Medicine Reports, 20, 73-80. https://doi.org/10.3892/mmr.2019.10220

8. http://nopr.niscair.res.in/handle/123456789/12736

9. https://doi.org/10.1016/S0944-7113(97)80033-5

10. Nalo Hamilton, Diana Marquez-Garban and Richard Pietras; DOI: 10.1158/1538-7445.AM2016-5077 Published July 2016

11. https://www.ncbi.nlm.nih.gov/pubmed/17178902

12. https://en.wikipedia.org/wiki/Clematis

13. Fungal symbionts produce prostaglandin E2 to promote their intestinal colonization; Tze Guan Tan, Ying;Shiang Lim, Alrina Tan, Royston Leong, Norman PavelkabioRxiv 477117; doi: https://doi.org/10.1101/477117

14. Rempel, Brian & Withers, Stephen. (2008). Covalent inhibitors of glycosidases and their applications in biochemistry and biology. Glycobiology. 18. 570-86. 10.1093/glycob/cwn041.

15. Yue Zhao, "The Oncogenic Functions of Nicotinic Acetylcholine Receptors," Journal of Oncology, vol. 2016, Article ID 9650481, 9 pages, 2016. https://doi.org/10.1155/2016/9650481

16. http://iv.iiarjournals.org/content/28/4/583.full.pdf+html

17. J Ethnopharmacol. 2016 Jun 20;186:305-310. doi: 10.1016/j.jep.2016.04.007. Epub 2016 Apr 13.

18. https://en.wikipedia.org/wiki/Goldenseal

19. Medicinal Plants of Australia: An Antipodean Apothecary by Cheryl Williams; p.n. 428.

20. https://www.ncbi.nlm.nih.gov/pubmed/19734580#

21. https://en.wikipedia.org/wiki/Ornithogalum_umbellatum

22. Antitumor effects of naturally occurring cardiac glycosides convallatoxin and peruvoside on human ER+ and triple-negative breast cancersdoi: 10.1038/cddiscovery.2017.9

23. https://www.sciencedirect.com/topics/pharmacology-toxicology-and-pharmaceutical-science/pokeweed-antivirus-protein

24. Antitumor Effects Of The Benzophenanthridine Alkaloid Sanguinarine: Evidence And Perspectives Https://Www.Ncbi.Nlm.Nih.Gov/Pmc/Articles/Pmc4714144/

25. Kalogris, Cristina &Garulli, Chiara &Pietrella, Lucia & Gambini, Valentina &Pucciarelli, Stefania & Lucci, Cristiano & Tilio, Martina & EléxpuruZabaleta, Maria & Bartolacci, Caterina &Andreani, Cristina & Giangrossi, Mara & Iezzi, Manuela & Belletti, Barbara & Marchini, Cristina & Amici, Augusto. (2014). Sanguinarine Suppresses Basal-Like Breast Cancer Growth through Dihydrofolate Reductase Inhibition. Biochemical Pharmacology. -. 10.1016/j.bcp.2014.05.014.

26. Sarsaparilla (Smilax Glabra Rhizome) Extract Inhibits Cancer Cell Growth By S Phase Arrest, Apoptosis, And Autophagy Via Redox-Dependent Erk1/2 Pathway Tiantian She, Like Qu, Lixin Wang, Xingxin Yang, Shuo Xu, Junnan Feng, Yujing Gao, Chuanke Zhao, Yong Han, Shaoqing Cai And Chengchao Shou

27. 2015 Jun;128:1-6. doi: 10.1016/j.chemosphere.2014.12.055. Epub 2015 Jan 17; Zearalenone and its metabolites in urine and breast cancer risk: a case-control study in Tunisia.; Belhassen H[1], Jiménez-Díaz I[2], Arrebola JP[3], Ghali R[1], Ghorbel H[1], Olea N[4], Hedili A[1].

28. Nakano, D., Ishitsuka, K., Kamikawa, M. et al. J Nat Med (2013) 67: 894. https://doi.org/10.1007/s11418-013-0747-2

29. https://www.botanica.ch/cms/dokumente/news/Documentation_Houseleek_V3.pdf

30. Medicinal significance, pharmacological activities, and analytical aspects of solasodine: A concise report of current scientific literatureIKanikaPatelaRaviB.SinghbDineshK.Patelchttps://doi.org/10.1016/S2221-6189(13)60106-7

31. Zarrinnahad, H., Mahmoodzadeh, A., Hamidi, M.P. et al. Int J Pept Res Ther (2018) 24: 563. https://doi.org/10.1007/s10989-017-9641-1

32. Lee, KS., Shin, JS. & Nam, KS. BiotechnolBioproc E (2011) 16: 987.; https://doi.org/10.1007/s12257-011-0226-0

33. Li, Fang & Huang, Qian & Chen, Jiang & Peng, Yuanlin&Roop, Dennis & Bedford, Joel & Li, Chuan-Yuan. (2010). Apoptotic Cells Activate the "Phoenix Rising" Pathway to Promote Wound Healing and Tissue Regeneration. Science signaling. 3. ra13. 10.1126/scisignal.2000634.

34. 10.1158/1538-7445.AM2018-3078 Published July 2018

35. 10.1186/s12935-019-0806-1

36. https://en.wikipedia.org/wiki/Common_toad

37. Gracheva, E. O., Ingolia, N. T., Kelly, Y. M., Cordero-Morales, J. F., Hollopeter, G., Chesler, A. T., ... Julius, D. (2010). Molecular basis of infrared detection by snakes. Nature, 464(7291), 1006–1011. doi:10.1038/nature08943

38. Toxins 2019, 11, 193; doi:10.3390/toxins11040193

39. http://www.jbc.org/content/243/6/1283.full.pdf

40. DOI 10.1016/j.chembiol.2003.11.010

41. http://ijpsr.com/bft-article/biochemical-composition-of-cuttle-fish-sepia-prabahari-ink-and-its-bioactive-properties-in-vitro/?view=fulltext

42. J Agric Food Chem. 2016 Jul 20;64(28):5759-66. doi: 10.1021/acs.jafc.6b01854. Epub 2016 Jul 6.

43. https://www.ncbi.nlm.nih.gov/pubmed/8877814; https://en.wikipedia.org/wiki/Chromatophore

44. Melatonin for The Prevention And Treatment Of Cancer Ya Li,1 Sha Li,#2 Yue Zhou,1 Xiao Meng,1 Jiao-Jiao Zhang,1 Dong-Ping Xu,1 and Hua-Bin Li#1,3;https://www.ncbi.nlm.nih.gov/pmc/articles/PMC5503661/

45. https://link.springer.com/article/10.1023/A:1015272401822

46. https://www.who.int/water_sanitation_health/diseases-risks/diseases/arsenicosis/en/

47. https://en.wikipedia.org/wiki/Gold

48. https://www.atsdr.cdc.gov/csem/csem.asp?csem=6&po=12

49. Epidemiology: November 2008 - Volume 19 - Issue 6 - p S110-S111;doi: 10.1097/01.ede.0000339863.17245.23

50. Kurdi M. S. (2016). Chronic fluorosis: The disease and its anaesthetic implications. Indian journal of anaesthesia, 60(3), 157–162. doi:10.4103/0019-5049.17786

51. fluoride-doped-hydroxyapatite-in-soft-tissues-and-cancer-a-literature-reviewhttps://www.researchgate.net/publication/272421380

52. Rappaport J. (2017). Changes in Dietary Iodine Explains Increasing Incidence of Breast Cancer with Distant Involvement in Young Women. Journal of Cancer, 8(2), 174–177. doi:10.7150/jca.17835

53. Dong, L., Lu, J., Zhao, B. et al. Review of the possible association between thyroid and breast carcinoma. World J SurgOnc 16, 130 (2018) doi:10.1186/s12957-018-1436-0

54. Mary Beth Martin, Ronald Reiter, Trung Pham, Yaniris R. Avellanet, Johanna Camara, Michael Lahm, Elisabeth Pentecost, Kiran Pratap, Brent A. Gilmore, ShailajaDivekar, Ross S. Dagata, Jaime L. Bull, Adriana Stoica, Estrogen-Like Activity of Metals in Mcf-7 Breast Cancer Cells, Endocrinology, Volume 144, Issue 6, 1 June 2003, Pages 2425–2436, https://doi.org/10.1210/en.2002-221054

55. Gaudet, H. M., Christensen, E., Conn, B., Morrow, S., Cressey, L., & Benoit, J. (2018). Methylmercury promotes breast cancer cell proliferation. Toxicology reports, 5, 579–584. doi:10.1016/j. toxrep.2018.05.002

56. https://www.ncbi.nlm.nih.gov/pubmed/28811684

57. Lead Exposure: A Contributing Cause of The Current Breast Cancer Epidemic In Nigerian Women; Https://Www.Ncbi.Nlm.Nih.Gov/ Pmc/Articles/Pmc2883097/

58. https://onlinelibrary.wiley.com/doi/pdf/10.1002/1097

59. C.Colin,et al;2017; Italy. DOI: 10.1051/radiopro/2017034

60. https://doi.org/10.1016/j.jaubas.2013.01.003

61. Chung GiLeeaHee-WeonLeeaByung-OhKimbDong-KwonRheeaSuhkneungPyoa https://doi.org/10.1016/j.jff.2015.03.017

62. https://www.ncbi.nlm.nih.gov/pubmed/30580607

63. https://www.mskcc.org/cancer-care/integrative-medicine/herbs/ astragalus

64. Chun, Jaemoo& Song, Kwangho& Kim, Yeong. (2018). Sesquiterpene lactonesenriched fraction of Inulahelenium L. induces apoptosis through inhibition of signal transducers and activators of transcription 3 signaling pathway in MDA-MB-231 breast cancer cells. Phytotherapy Research. 32. 10.1002/ptr.6189.

65. Thakur, Ajay. (2011). Juglone: A therapeutic phytochemical from Juglans L. J. Med. Plants Res. 5. 5324-5330.

66. Zhou and Lu, 2016; Russo Spena et al., 2018

67. https://link.springer.com/article/10.1007/s11655-011-0819-7

68. https://www.sciencedirect.com/science/article/abs/pii/ S0031942213002045

69. www.bmjournal.in BM/Vol.4/August 2013/bm- 29205121813

70. Nisreen Al-Bayati /J. Pharm. Sci. & Res. Vol. 10(8), 2018, 2014-2016